Jeffrey R. Guss, MD
Jack Drescher, MD
Editors

D0706323

Addictions in the Gay and Lesbian Community

Addictions in the Gay and Lesbian Community
has been co-published simultaneously as *Journal
of Gay & Lesbian Psychotherapy,* Volume 3,
Numbers 3/4 2000.

*Pre-Publication
REVIEWS,
COMMENTARIES,
EVALUATIONS . . .*

"**W**e can learn a great deal from emerging areas of psychiatry, and this unique book certainly fills this bill. It is a cogent study at the interface of substance abuse problems and the culture of the gay and lesbian community. The issues it presents need to be understood by thoughtful clinicians and by students of this important and vibrant American minority. We have in this book a sophisticated perspective on the social, psychological and treatment questions raised by its title."

Marc Galanter, MD
*Professor of Psychiatry
and Director
Division of Alcoholism
and Drug Abuse
NYU Medical Center
New York*

"**A**ddictions in the Gay and Lesbian Community* is a unique, in-depth, excellent reference to improve substance abuse diagnosis, for all health professionals, in all general and specialty medical fields and in all areas of mental health and substance abuse fields for more appropriate treatment as well.

Well written chapters by all the contributors highlight the necessary common and unique specifics of identifying gay, lesbian, bisexual and transgender patients with substance abuse and psychiatric disorders, at increased rates, often because of painful and stereotypic experiences from their earliest years in homes, schools and among peers.

Chapters such as treating professionals who are also gay, lesbian, bisexual and transgender and whose intellect and education enable them to use self-defeating defenses, to one on needs for special gay sensitive substance abuse treatment programs, and unique issues in psychoanalytic, psychodynamic and cognitive-behavioral treatment issues will be invaluable to all readers, including patients, to increase understanding and thus improve earlier diagnosis and more appropriate treatment with the likelihood of more successful outcomes. This important edited volume, by Dr. Guss and Dr. Drescher is unique in topics included and its potential usefulness for all readers; it is definitely well worth reading and rereading, and even sharing with the public, including teachers, the legal system and all front-line community leaders."

Leah J. Dickstein, MD, MA
Professor
Department of Psychiatry
and Behavioral Siciences
University of Louisville
School of Medicine

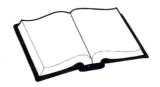

More pre-publication
REVIEWS, COMMENTARIES, EVALUATIONS . . .

"**T**his is a stimulating and useful book on an important topic. Gay and lesbian substance abuses, largely ignored a generation or two ago, are common, destructive, and too often avoided or denied.

This book is clear, fairly short, and efficient. It is practical and timely, combining helpful biopsychosocial theory with social awareness, psychological subtlety, and clinical balance.

Alcohol remains a deservedly major focus, but there is also attention to circuit party designer drugs, with their cute initials, like the initials on designer clothes but slightly more lethal.

Reading this book should interest and help most of all mental health professionals in all disciplines, not just addiction specialists."

Lawrence Hartmann, MD
Past President
American Psychiatric Association

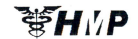

The Haworth Medical Press
An Imprint of
The Haworth Press, Inc.

Addictions in the Gay and Lesbian Community

Addictions in the Gay and Lesbian Community has been co-published simultaneously as *Journal of Gay & Lesbian Psychotherapy* Volume 3, Numbers 3/4 2000.

The *Journal of Gay & Lesbian Psychotherapy* Monographic "Separates"

Below is a list of "separates," which in serials librarianship means a special issue simultaneously published as a special journal issue or double-issue *and* as a "separate" hardbound monograph. (This is a format which we also call a "DocuSerial.")

"Separates" are published because specialized libraries or professionals may wish to purchase a specific thematic issue by itself in a format which can be separately cataloged and shelved, as opposed to purchasing the journal on an on-going basis. Faculty members may also more easily consider a "separate" for classroom adoption.

"Separates" are carefully classified separately with the major book jobbers so that the journal tie-in can be noted on new book order slips to avoid duplicate purchasing.

You may wish to visit Haworth's website at . . .

http://www.HaworthPress.com

. . . to search our online catalog for complete tables of contents of these separates and related publications.

You may also call 1-800-HAWORTH (outside US/Canada: 607-722-5857), or Fax: 1-800-895-0582 (outside US/Canada: 607-771-0012), or e-mail at:

getinfo@haworthpressinc.com

Addictions in the Gay and Lesbian Community, edited by Jeffrey R. Guss, MD, and Jack Drescher, MD (Vol. 3, No. 3/4, 2000). *Explores the unique clinical considerations involved in addiction treatment for gay men and lesbians, groups that reportedly use and abuse alcohol and substances at higher rates than the general population.*

Addictions
in the Gay and Lesbian
Community

Jeffrey R. Guss, MD
Jack Drescher, MD
Editors

Addictions in the Gay and Lesbian Community has been co-published simultaneously as *Journal of Gay & Lesbian Psychotherapy*, Volume 3, Numbers 3/4 2000.

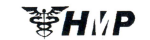

The Haworth Medical Press
An Imprint of
The Haworth Press, Inc.
New York • London • Oxford

Published by

The Haworth Medical Press®, 10 Alice Street, Binghamton, NY 13904-1580, USA

The Haworth Medical Press® is an imprint of The Haworth Press, Inc., 10 Alice Street, Binghamton, NY 13904-1580 USA.

Addictions in the Gay and Lesbian Community has been co-published simultaneously as *Journal of Gay & Lesbian Psychotherapy* ™, Volume 3, Numbers 3/4 2000.

© 2000 by The Haworth Press, Inc. All rights reserved. No part of this work may be reproduced or utilized in any form or by any means, electronic or mechanical, including photocopying, microfilm and recording, or by any information storage and retrieval system, without permission in writing from the publisher. Printed in the United States of America.

The development, preparation, and publication of this work has been undertaken with great care. However, the publisher, employees, editors, and agents of The Haworth Press and all imprints of The Haworth Press, Inc., including The Haworth Medical Press® and Pharmaceutical Products Press®, are not responsible for any errors contained herein or for consequences that may ensue from use of materials or information contained in this work. Opinions expressed by the author(s) are not necessarily those of The Haworth Press, Inc.

Library of Congress Cataloging-in-Publication Data

Addictions in the gay and lesbian community / Jeffrey R. Guss, Jack Drescher, editors.
    p. cm.
    ". . . has been co-published simultaneously as Journal of gay & lesbian psychotherapy."
    Includes bibliographical references and index.
    ISBN 0-7890-1037-2 (alk. paper) – ISBN 0-7890-1038-0 (alk. paper)
    1. Gays–Substance use. 2. Substance abuse–Treatment. I. Guss, Jeffrey R. II. Drescher, Jack, 1951- III. Journal of gay & lesbian psychotherapy.
RC564.5.G39 A33 2000
616.86′0086′64–dc21
                                      00-046152

Indexing, Abstracting & Website/Internet Coverage

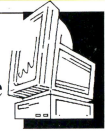

This section provides you with a list of major indexing & abstracting services. That is to say, each service began covering this periodical during the year noted in the right column. Most Websites which are listed below have indicated that they will either post, disseminate, compile, archive, cite or alert their own Website users with research-based content from this work. (This list is as current as the copyright date of this publication.)

Abstracting, Website/Indexing Coverage .... Year When Coverage Began

- *Abstracts in Anthropology* 1991
- *Academic Index (on-line)* 1992
- *BUBL Information Service: An Internet-based Information Service for the UK higher education community <URL: http://bubl.ac.uk/>* 1995
- *CNPIEC Reference Guide: Chinese National Directory of Foreign Periodicals* 1995
- *Contemporary Women's Issues* 1998
- *Expanded Academic Index* 1995
- *Family Studies Database (online and CD/ROM)* 1998
- *Family Violence & Sexual Assault Institute* 1992
- *FINDEX <www.publist.com>* 1999
- *Gay & Lesbian Abstracts* 1999
- *GenderWatch <www.slinfo.com>* 1999
- *HOMODOK/"Relevant" Bibliographic database, Documentation Centre for Gay & Lesbian Studies, University of Amsterdam (selective printed abstracts in "Homologie" and bibliographic computer databases covering cultural, historical, social and political aspects of gay & lesbian topics)* 1995

(continued)

- *Index to Periodical Articles Related to Law* **1993**
- *Leeds Medical Information* **1995**
- *MasterFILE: updated database from EBSCO Publishing* **1998**
- *Mental Health Abstracts (online through DIALOG)* **1993**
- *MLA International Bibliography (available in print,*
  on CD-ROM and Internet) **1995**
- *Periodcial Abstracts, Research II (broad coverage*
  indexing & abstracting data-base from University
  Microfilms International (UMI) **1993**
- *Referativnyi Zhurnal (Abstracts Journal of the All-Russian*
  Institute of Scientific and Technical Information) **1991**
- *Sage Family Studies Abstracts (SFSA)* **1993**
- *Social Services Abstracts <www.csa.com>* **1991**
- *Social Work Abstracts* **1993**
- *Sociological Abstracts (SA) <www.csa.com>* **1991**
- *Studies on Women Abstracts* **1993**
- *Violence and Abuse Abstracts: A Review of Current*
  Literature on Interpersonal Violence (VAA) **1995**

Special Bibliographic Notes related to special journal issues
(separates) and indexing/abstracting:

- indexing/abstracting services in this list will also cover material in any "separate" that is co-published simultaneously with Haworth's special thematic journal issue or DocuSerial. Indexing/abstracting usually covers material at the article/chapter level.
- monographic co-editions are intended for either non-subscribers or libraries which intend to purchase a second copy for their circulating collections.
- monographic co-editions are reported to all jobbers/wholesalers/approval plans. The source journal is listed as the "series" to assist the prevention of duplicate purchasing in the same manner utilized for books-in-series.
- to facilitate user/access services all indexing/abstracting services are encouraged to utilize the co-indexing entry note indicated at the bottom of the first page of each article/chapter/contribution.
- this is intended to assist a library user of any reference tool (whether print, electronic, online, or CD-ROM) to locate the monographic version if the library has purchased this version but not a subscription to the source journal.
- individual articles/chapters in any Haworth publication are also available through the Haworth Document Delivery Service (HDDS).

Addictions
in the Gay and Lesbian
Community

CONTENTS

Introduction   1
    Jeffrey R. Guss, MD

OVERVIEWS AND EMPIRICAL STUDY

Substance Abuse, Internalized Homophobia, and Gay Men
    and Lesbians: Psychodynamic Issues and Clinical
    Implications   5
    Robert Paul Cabaj, MD

The Prevalence of Alcoholism and Feelings of Alienation
    in Lesbian and Heterosexual Women   25
    Carrie Jaffe, PhD
    Pauline Rose Clance, PhD
    Margaret F. Nichols, PhD
    James G. Emshoff, PhD

Gay Men, Lesbians and Substances of Abuse and the "Club
    and Circuit Party Scene": What Clinicians Should Know   37
    David McDowell, MD

SPECIAL POPULATIONS AND TREATMENT SETTINGS

Treating Gay, Lesbian, Bisexual and Transgender Professionals
    with Addictive Disease   59
    Penelope P. Ziegler, MD

Gay Teens and Substance Use Disorders: Assessment
    and Treatment   69
    Eva D. Olson, MD

The Importance of Specialized Treatment Programs for Lesbian
    and Gay Patients   81
    Daniel Hicks, MD

OFFICE-BASED ADDICTION TREATMENT

A Memoir of Homosexuality, Psychiatry, Chemical
    Dependence, Depression and Recovery: Confessions
    of a Social Activist   95
        Anonymous

Sex Like You Can't Even Imagine: "Crystal," Crack
    and Gay Men   105
        Jeffrey R. Guss, MD

Psychoanalytic and Behavioral Approaches to Drug-Related
    Sexual Risk Taking: A Preliminary Conceptual
    and Clinical Integration   123
        David G. Ostrow, MD, PhD
        R. Dennis Shelby, PhD

Sexual Compulsivity in Gay Men from a Jungian Perspective   141   ⌲
        John A. Gosling, MD

Reification and the Ecstasy of the Chelsea Boy   169
        Stephen Hartman, PhD

Index   187

ABOUT THE EDITORS

Jeffrey R. Guss, MD, is Clinical Assistant Professor of Psychiatry at the New York University School of Medicine. He is a Candidate at the New York University Postdoctoral Program in Psychotherapy and Psychoanalysis, and maintains a private practice in analytic psychotherapy as well as the treatment of addictive disorders. He is on the Editorial Board of the *Journal of Gay & Lesbian Psychotherapy*. He has served as Unit Chief of the primary teaching setting for Fellows in the NYU Division of Alcoholism and Drug Abuse at Bellevue Hospital. Prior to this, Dr. Guss developed outpatient treatment programs for addictive disorders at New York Hospital-Cornell Medical Center-Westchester Division in White Plains, New York, and the Ann Arbor Veteran's Administration Medical Center in Ann Arbor, Michigan, where he also served as Director of Resident Education.

Jack Drescher, MD, Editor-in-Chief of the *Journal of Gay & Lesbian Psychotherapy*, is Supervisor of Psychoanalysis and Faculty Member at the William Alanson White Psychoanalytic Institute and Clinical Assistant Professor of Psychiatry at SUNY–Brooklyn. He Chairs the Committee on Human Sexuality of the Group for the Advancement of Psychiatry (GAP) and is a member of the American College of Psychiatrists. Author of *Psychoanalytic Therapy and the Gay Man* (1998, The Analytic Press), Dr. Drescher is in full-time private practice in New York City.

ALL HAWORTH MEDICAL PRESS BOOKS
AND JOURNALS ARE PRINTED
ON CERTIFIED ACID-FREE PAPER

Introduction

I eagerly anticipated my first psychoanalytic psychotherapy patient as part of my psychiatry residency at the University of Michigan in the late 1970s. That part of our program was run like an analytic institute, with patients, carefully chosen by a senior clinician, who were deemed ready for treatment three times per week. I secretly hoped mine would neither be gay nor have problems with homosexuality. I was in the process of coming out to myself, but was still in the closet at work, and I know I wouldn't be able to untangle my own anxieties from those I was to treat.

It was an anxious time for me. During my adolescence, I had read the frightening and infuriating books of Bieber, Socarides, Ovesey and Bergler, and the prospect of finding a stable, safe therapeutic position for myself as both therapist and supervisee seemed impossible. Yet while these four might have been writing from clinical experience, I knew they were doing so as outsiders and, despite all their protestations to the contrary, with a certain hostility. It took several years for me to understand that whatever they claimed might "cause" homosexuality reflected their own theoretical and personal biases, lacking any objective authority.

As I came out of the closet, I met more gay people and read what seemed like radical works by gay psychiatrists and activists. I was utterly thrilled when I walked into my first AGLP Opening Reception at the APA Annual Meeting. Slowly, I discovered the difference between the view from the inside and the outside. Once Kenneth Lewes' groundbreaking book *The Psychoanalytic Theory of Male Homosexuality* was published, the "authority" of those abovenamed analytic writers was exploded from the inside with great power.

Indeed, the reality of gay men and women writing about ourselves has

[Haworth co-indexing entry note]: "Introduction." Guss, Jeffrey R. Co-published simultaneously in *Journal of Gay & Lesbian Psychotherapy* (The Haworth Medical Press, an imprint of The Haworth Press, Inc.) Vol. 3, No. 3/4, 2000, pp. 1-3; and: *Addictions in the Gay and Lesbian Community* (ed: Jeffrey R. Guss, and Jack Drescher) The Haworth Medical Press, an imprint of The Haworth Press, Inc., 2000, pp. 1-3. Single or multiple copies of this article are available from The Haworth Document Delivery Service [1-800-342-9678, 9:00 a.m. - 5:00 p.m. (EST). E-mail address: getinfo@haworthpressinc.com].

© 2000 by The Haworth Press, Inc. All rights reserved.

profoundly changed the theories we use and the ways we conduct clinical practice. This change can be seen in every article written for this publication. It was a pleasure to watch this work take shape as the authors contributed articles written from their own experiences treating or studying gay and lesbian patients with addictive disorders.

The work begins with an overview by Bob Cabaj, well known in our community for his numerous contributions to the field. Carrie Jaffe and her collaborators compare lesbian and heterosexual women in terms of prevalence of alcoholism and feelings of alienation with some surprising results. (The *Journal of Gay & Lesbian Psychotherapy* wishes to acknowledge Laura Post, MD's contribution to the editorial process in the acceptance of this paper.) David McDowell provides a comprehensive overview of club drugs, including historical, pharmacological and clinical perspectives. Two special populations within the gay and lesbian community are discussed, professionals and adolescents. Penelope Ziegler shares her experience treating gay, lesbian and bisexual doctors and nurses; Eva Olson writes about adolescents, describing the ways that evaluation and treatment must be modified for this population. Dan Hicks describes a treatment setting designed exclusively for gay, lesbian and bisexual patients. Anonymous has written a moving essay on his experience as a gay physician, political activist, in recovery from addiction and depression. His anonymity is required according to the principles of Alcoholics Anonymous rather than a personal need for secrecy. The remaining articles describe clinical approaches useful in more traditional office-based treatment settings. Jeffrey Guss has written about the treatment of gay men addicted to stimulant drugs and sex. David Ostrow and R. Dennis Shelby provide an integration of psychoanalytic and cognitive behavioral approaches in the treatment of gay men. John Gosling and his patient describe the experience of sexual addiction and recovery from the perspective of Jungian psychotherapy. Stephen Hartman concludes the work, utilizing a post-structural perspective to explore the inner world of the addicted "Chelsea Boy" seeking reification.

Numerous books have been published about addiction and recovery for the gay, lesbian and bisexual community. They often refer to the themes that are recurrent in these articles: homophobia, shame, secrecy, and loneliness. I hope this collection will be a useful addition to the growing body of writing on this topic, written by clinicians from the inside.

Jeffrey R. Guss, MD

REFERENCES

Bieber, I., Dain, H., Dince, P., Drellich, M., Grand, H., Gundlach, R., Dremer, M., Rifkin, A., Wilbur, C., and Bieber T. (1962), *Homosexuality: A Psychoanalytic Study*. New York: Basic Books.

Bergler, E. (1956), *Homosexuality: Disease or Way of Life*. New York: Hill and Wang.

Lewes, K. (1988), *The Psychoanalytic Theory of Male Homosexuality*. New York: Simon and Schuster.

Ovesey, L. (1969), *Homosexuality and Pseudohomosexuality*. New York: Science House.

Socarides, C. (1968), *The Overt Homosexual*. New York: Grune and Stratton.

OVERVIEWS AND EMPIRICAL STUDY

Substance Abuse, Internalized Homophobia, and Gay Men and Lesbians: Psychodynamic Issues and Clinical Implications

Robert Paul Cabaj, MD

SUMMARY. Gay men and lesbians reportedly use and abuse alcohol and substances at rates higher than the general population. This higher rate has been questioned, but, whether gay men and lesbians have more use and abuse or not, unique clinical considerations are involved in addiction treatment for gay men and lesbians. The psychodynamic factors that contribute to the creation and powerful influence of internalized homophobia for gay men and lesbians can explain the predisposition to substance use and abuse. Parents may not be able to acknowledge or reward the differences that may be apparent in the pre-homosexual child. The child will learn to hide or dissociate from those differences. In addition, the psychology of difference, that is, learning how to live with and accept things about one's

Dr. Robert Paul Cabaj is affiliated with San Mateo Mental Health Services, 225 37th Avenue, San Mateo, CA 94403.

[Haworth co-indexing entry note]: "Substance Abuse, Internalized Homophobia, and Gay Men and Lesbians: Psychodynamic Issues and Clinical Implications." Cabaj, Robert Paul. Co-published simultaneously in *Journal of Gay & Lesbian Psychotherapy* (The Haworth Medical Press, an imprint of The Haworth Press, Inc.) Vol. 3, No. 3/4, 2000, pp. 5-24; and: *Addictions in the Gay and Lesbian Community* (ed: Jeffrey R. Guss, and Jack Drescher) The Haworth Medical Press, an imprint of The Haworth Press, Inc., 2000, pp. 5-24. Single or multiple copies of this article are available from The Haworth Document Delivery Service [1-800-342-9678, 9:00 a.m. - 5:00 p.m. (EST). E-mail address: getinfo@haworthpressinc.com].

© 2000 by The Haworth Press, Inc. All rights reserved.

self that are different from the majority, will contribute to further denial and dissociation from true feelings and needs. Substance use allows the expression of suppressed and repressed desires and needs and facilitates denial and dissociation. Gay men and lesbians may find the comfort in using drugs and alcohol leads to increased use, abuse, and possible dependency. Treatment of gay men and lesbians with substance use disorders will need to address the internalized homophobia as part of the recovery process. Traditional psychotherapy will not be helpful while the individual is actively drinking or drugging but supportive therapy can be quite helpful until the individual is in recovery. Psychotherapy then can be used to help accept and integrate a gay or lesbian identity and help support relapse prevention. *[Article copies available for a fee from The Haworth Document Delivery Service: 1-800-342-9678. E-mail address: <getinfo@haworthpress inc.com> Website: <http://www.HaworthPress.com>]*

KEYWORDS. Homosexuality, substance use disorders, homophobia, addiction treatment, psychotherapy, psychology of difference, dissociation

The mental health literature on substance use and abuse among gay men and lesbians is extensive and continues to grow. The focus of most of the literature is on the extent of the use or abuse, the effect substance use has on gay people, the association with exposure to the Human Immunodeficiency Virus (HIV) associated with Acquired Immune Deficiency Syndrome (AIDS), and clinical interventions for gay people. There has been little written on the psychodynamic, psychological, and emotional issues related to substance use and abuse for gay men and lesbians, and little on the role of psychotherapy with substance using/abusing gay men and lesbians. Less studied as well are substance use and abuse among bisexual men and women or among transgender persons. This article will review some of the literature, describe some of the psychodynamic issues, and explore the clinical implications for gay men and lesbians who use and abuse substances.

EPIDEMIOLOGY

There is no solid agreement about the amount of alcohol and other substances used or the incidence of substance abuse in the gay and lesbian population. Most studies (Saghir and Robbins, 1973; Diamond and Wilsnack, 1978; Lohrenz et al., 1978; Lewis, Saghir, and Robins, 1982; Beatty, 1983; Mosbacher, 1988; Pillard, 1988; McKirman and Peterson, 1989a), reports (Fifield, de Crescenzo, and Latham, 1975; Lesbian and Gay Substance Abuse Planning Group, 1991), reviews of surveys (Weinberg and Williams, 1974;

Morales and Graves, 1983), and the experiences of most clinicians working with gay men and lesbians (Finnegan and McNally, 1987; Cabaj, 1997) estimate an incidence of substance abuse of all types at approximately 30%, with ranges of 28-35%. This estimate contrasts with an incidence of 10-12% for the general population.

A careful review of each report, however, demonstrates significant and persistent methodological problems, ranging from poor or absent control groups, unrepresentative population samples (some studies gathered subjects only from gay and lesbian bars), to a failure to use uniform definitions of substance abuse or of homosexuality itself. One major problem in studies that attempt to look at prevalence and/or incidence of substance use or abuse amongst gay and lesbian people is the limited data on the actual numbers of gay people. Due to stigma and other fears, gay people may not be forthcoming about their sexual orientation in surveys and studies.

Nonetheless, no matter where the sample was taken–urban or rural, various socioeconomic settings, in the United States or other countries--the rates are strikingly uniform, though some variations are reported. For example, Stall and Wiley (1988), using very simple screening questions, note greater substance use but no greater alcohol use amongst gay men as compared to heterosexual men in San Francisco. McKirman and Peterson (1989a) report that heavy alcohol use was not greater for gay men and lesbians compared to heterosexuals sampled, but did note that there were fewer gay and lesbian alcohol abstainers and a greater number of gay and lesbian moderate alcohol users.

Currently, no study specifically focuses on the drug or alcohol use of bisexual men or women, though many such people are included in some of the studies described above. Also, there are as yet no studies focused on transgender people's substance abuse.

Alcohol abuse has been the primary focus of most studies, with no specific studies of injecting drug use (IDU) and the gay population currently available. The Center for Disease Control's (CDC) quarterly report on AIDS and HIV infections clearly indicates a subgroup of IDU gay and bisexual men, and one of the routes of HIV infection for lesbians is injecting drug use (CDC, 1998).

PREDISPOSITION FOR SUBSTANCE ABUSE

Many factors contribute to the prominent role of substance use and abuse in gay men and lesbians. At one point, American psychoanalytic psychiatry, for years focused on the etiology of male homosexuality, even postulated that homosexuality was a cause of alcoholism (Israelstam and Lambert, 1983). Since homosexuality, repressed or not, does not cause alcoholism (Israelstam and Lambert, 1986)–indeed, alcoholism and substance abuse are not "caused" by any psychodynamic or personality factor alone–other factors must be examined, the two most important being: (1) genetic and biological contributions and (2) the psychological effects of heterosexism and homophobia, both external and internal.

In looking at the etiology of sexual orientation, most new research indicates that a homosexual orientation is not learned and is not a result of any family or social pattern. There is continuing and growing evidence that homosexual orientation may have genetic, biological, and biochemical components (Pillard, Poumadere, and Carretta, 1982; Pillard and Weinrich, 1986; Bailey and Pillard, 1991; Bailey and Benishay, 1993; Pillard, 1988). Some studies of familial patterns (Pillard, Poumadere, and Carretta, 1982; Pillard, 1988) point out that gay men have a greater than normal chance of having an alcoholic father.

New research continues to support the genetic, biological, and biochemical contributions to substance use disorders. It is possible that the genetic materials for sexual orientation and substance abuse are chromosomally linked–explaining the possible higher incidence in the gay population. It is clear, however, from several studies that the genetics of male and female homosexuality are different, with different familial patterns (Bell and Weinberg, 1978; Bell, Weinberg, and Hammersmith, 1981; Pillard, 1988); yet, rates of substance abuse are the same for gay men and lesbians.

Most societies or cultures in turmoil, or undergoing social change, have higher rates of alcoholism (Cassel, 1976; Vaillant, 1983). Gay men and lesbians have faced great societal prohibitions, not only against the expression of their sexual feelings and behavior, but also against their very existence. Legal prohibitions on homosexual behavior, overt discrimination, and the failure of society to accept or even acknowledge gay people have tended to limit the types of social outlets available to gay men and lesbians to bars, private homes, or clubs where alcohol and other drugs often play a prominent role. Often, the role models for many young gay men and lesbians just coming out are gay people using alcohol and other drugs, met at bars or parties. Continuing societal anti-gay bias, as well as the impact of HIV on gay men and lesbians, further add to the stress (Israelstam and Lambert, 1989; McKirman and Peterson, 1989b).

Even while gay men and lesbians have created alternatives and discovered additional ways to meet and express themselves, a major stumbling block still exists because of societal homophobia–the fear and hatred of gay men, lesbians, and homosexuality itself. Homophobia is the major force that gay people must deal with in our society, both internalized, that is, within the individual, incorporated by societal norms, and external, as expressed by societal forces directly (Weinberg, 1972; De Cecco, 1984; Cabaj, 1985; Forstein, 1988; Herek, 1996).

Anti-gay bias is found in every sector in our society: legal, medical, scientific, religious, political, social, educational, and judicial. The ever increasing violent and legal attacks on gay men and lesbians, from verbal threats to outright physical attacks and murder, are usually fueled by such anti-gay bias (Klinger and Stein, 1996). Exploration of the links between the use or abuse of substances and gay or lesbian identity formation may help explain the process by which many gay people turn to alcohol and drug use.

All gay people have internalized homophobia, having been brought up in a homophobic society that either tends to promote prejudicial myths about gay people or negates the existence of gay people in general. The coming out process may be delayed or very difficult to negotiate depending on the intensity of internalized homophobia. The gay person may believe, depending on familial, religious, cultural, and local societal influences, that homosexuality is a sin, an illness, unnatural, evil, or will only lead to sadness, loneliness, and isolation. It is a normal developmental step for most gay men and lesbians to wish they were not homosexual, depending on the effects of the above influences.

Identity development as a gay or lesbian person, and the concomitant coming out phenomena, is a long and complex process that continues throughout the entire life cycle; it has been formulated in various ways (de Monteflores and Schultz, 1978; Cass, 1996; McDonald, 1982; Hanley-Hackenbruck, 1988; Coleman, 1982). The easiest way to conceptualize coming out may be to view it as a series of steps an individual negotiates at his or her own time and pace, with periodic steps forward and backward. The individual must first become aware of his or her own sexual orientation as different from that of the majority. The next step is to accept the awareness and to begin to integrate it into a self-concept and to grapple with the negative feelings that may be associated. Next, the individual may choose to act on these feelings, although some people with strong homoerotic feelings never engage in sex with others of the same sex. Finally, the person makes a series of life-long decisions about whether to let others know and whom to let know, such as friends, family, work colleagues and peers, teachers, and medical providers. Some gay people only come out to selected people, some not to everyone at once. Some may come out, then deny it later or not continue to let new friends or people at new workplaces know. The extreme difficulty some gay men and women have in coming out and integrating sexuality and personal identity, facing possible rejection, can help explain the need to develop a false but acceptable self, as described above.

Developmental Issues

Reviewing the developmental issues for gay men and lesbians demonstrates that many of the clinical issues that are unique are a result of the adjustment to a minority sexual orientation and not due to any psychopathology associated with the orientation itself. There are three major tasks that gay men and lesbians must undertake that heterosexual people need not: first, recognition that there is indeed something "different" about them, that sense of difference usually preceding an awareness of sexual and affectionate feelings different from the majority; second, "coming out," that is, acknowledgement first to themselves and then eventually to others that they have a different sexual orientation; and third, healing the damage of internalized homophobia with possible confrontation of heterosexism and anti-gay bias experienced in coming out to others and living in the world as openly gay or lesbian.

The literature on the psychology of difference is very helpful in understanding some basic developmental issues. Learning to live in a society that does not accept difference readily shapes the identity development of many children who will grow up to be gay or lesbian. de Monteflores (1986) in particular describes how difficult it is to grow up different. Whereas a person of color cannot hide skin color, and the difference is obvious to all, a person with a homosexual orientation, while aware of being different, may not be recognized as different by anyone else. In a society that promotes and supports heterosexuality, the sense of difference in these children may be confusing and alienating, leading to social isolation and denial of natural feeling. Isay (1989) notes that the boy who will grow up to be gay may act or behave in such a way as to make some heterosexual fathers uncomfortable and lead to the fathers' withdrawal. For those children who are gender discordant in behavior, profound damage to self-esteem and other aspects of the personality may result from being shunned, humiliated, and derided by their peers (Hanson and Hartmann, 1996).

The vast majority of parents are heterosexual and raise their children either assuming that they will be heterosexual, or not thinking about their sexual orientation at all. For the pre-gay or pre-lesbian child (that is, the child who will grow up to be gay or lesbian), exposure to such non-confirming behavior and parental expectations enhances the feelings of being different. As a coping mechanism, pre-gay or pre-lesbian children commonly learn to disconnect and dissociate from their true selves and sexual orientation and adapt to parental expectations by creating and presenting a false self that is not a genuine reflection of the true self. For the gay child, that awareness of being "different"–having affectional and sexual longings that are different from the others around him–is usually evident quite early in life, especially in men. Dissociation and denial become major defenses.

As is true for all children, the child who will grow up to be gay or lesbian wants the love and acceptance of his or her parents and other caregivers. If the parents cannot respond to or give support for what is unfamiliar or uncomfortable for them, they will either ignore those attributes of the child that suggest difference, or try to change them. This rejection and criticism, both real and perceived, leads to pain, denial, isolation, and fear.

This process of ignoring may be quite subtle, a process of neglect poignantly described by the Swiss psychoanalyst Alice Miller in her early works (1981, 1984). Miller's description of parents who form, and deform, the emotional lives of their talented or different children has strong parallels with the development of many gay children. Parental reactions help to shape and validate the expression of the needs and longings of their children; parents more frequently reward what is familiar and acceptable to them and tend to discourage or de-emphasize behavior and needs they do not value or understand.

Harm occurs when a parent is too depressed, preoccupied, narcissistic, or under the influence of drugs or alcohol, to respond to the actual needs and wants of the child. Children eventually learn to behave the way parents expect, and to hide or deny the longings or needs that are not rewarded.

Dissociation and denial may become major defenses in the personality structure of such children, since they learn early that their feelings and needs are not acceptable and must be hidden and suppressed. Thus, the psychological effects of being different profoundly shape the way sexual identity develops and is then expressed by gay people as they emerge from childhood. In addition, these children are unlikely to have clear and positive role models of gay adults available to them; for example, the sexual orientation and relationship status of gay and lesbian teachers are rarely revealed, and there is little positive media attention given to gay men and lesbians. In adolescence, sexual feelings emerge with greater urgency, but there is rarely any context or permission for their expression. Adolescents in particular often reject and isolate those who are different and encourage conformity, which further supports denial and suppression of the emerging homosexual feelings. As a result, the adolescent who is gay or lesbian may even further split off awareness of affect and behavior related to his or her homosexuality (Martin, 1982).

When adolescents who have disconnected themselves from any awareness of their homosexual feelings begin to recognize the source of their sense of difference, they may work even harder to suppress these feelings by isolating themselves and avoiding situations that may stir up their longings. Some of these youths may devote extraordinary energy to academic or career success to cover up their underlying shame and sense of being defective; others may become depressed, isolated, guarded, and lonely, expecting to be rejected and ignored if their true feelings were revealed (Hetrick and Martin, 1987). Often these young people become ashamed not only of their sexual feelings, but also of their bodies, their social interactions, and other aspects of themselves. While not all gay men and lesbians have the same degree of difficulty traversing childhood and integrating an often stigmatized sexual identity into a healthy personality structure, most will show some residual signs of this difficult developmental path. For example, a sense of shame about being gay–a form of internalized homophobia–may persist.

Substance use serves as an easy relief, can provide acceptance, and, more importantly, mirrors the "comforting" dissociation developed in childhood. Alcohol and other drugs cause dissociation from feelings and anxiety, mimicking the emotional state many gay people had to develop in childhood to survive. These "symptom-relieving" aspects help fight the effects of homophobia; it can allow "forbidden" behavior, allow social comfort in bars or other unfamiliar social settings, and provide comfort through the dissociative state itself. Some gay people cannot imagine socializing without alcohol or other mood-altering substance. Many men had their early homosexual sexual experiences while drinking or being high. This association is a very powerful behavioral link–the "pleasure" and release of substance use and the pleasure and release of sex–and very difficult to change or "unlink" later in life.

For gay men especially, sex and intimacy are often split off or dissociated from one another. Again, substance use may allow acting on feelings long suppressed or denied, but also mirrors the dissociative experience and makes it harder to integrate intimacy and love. Sex and/or substances provide an instantly gratifying relief or satisfaction of longings and needs, decreasing the more complex challenges of love and intimacy.

For many men and women, this linking of substance use and sexuality persists and may become part of the coming-out process and the formation of a social and personal identity. Many gay people continue to feel self-hatred; the use of mood-altering substances temporarily relieves, but then reinforces this self-loathing in the drug withdrawal period. Alcohol and many other drugs can cause depression, leading to a further worsening of self-esteem.

Because of the childhood experience of not being acknowledged or accepted for who he or she is, gay men and lesbians are especially sensitive to rejection, and may expect it or even seek it out unconsciously; substance use helps many brace themselves for rejection by others, and may make "living in the closet," with its built in need for denial and dissociation, easier or even possible. Substance use seems to serve as an easy relief from negative feelings, can provide a degree of social acceptance, and, more importantly, reinforces what has come to be a comforting dissociation developed in childhood. The symptom-relieving aspects of substance use can serve to disinhibit what are experienced as forbidden behaviors, provide comfort through the familiar experiences of numbness, dissociation, and isolation of feelings.

The internal state that accompanies internalized homophobia and that occurs with substance abuse are very similar, the "dual oppression" of homophobia and substance abuse (Finnegan and McNally, 1987). The following traits can be seen in both: denial; fear, anxiety, and paranoia; anger and rage; guilt; self-pity; depression, with helplessness, hopelessness, and power-lessness; self-deception and development of a false self; passivity and the feeling of being a victim; inferiority and low self-esteem; self-loathing; isolation, alienation, and feeling alone, misunderstood, or unique; and fragmentation and confusion. These close similarities make it very difficult for gay men or lesbians who cannot accept their sexual orientation to recognize or successfully treat their substance abuse.

PSYCHOTHERAPY: SPECIAL CONSIDERATIONS

Gay men and lesbians seek mental health services for the same reasons anyone might–help with emotional and social problems, treatment for mental illness, treatment for substance abuse, couples therapy, family therapy, and so on–but there are some special considerations in working with this population. The developmental issues unique to forming a gay or lesbian identity need to be considered in any psychotherapy or counseling. The way a gay man or lesbian has dealt with his or her internalized homophobia and how he or she has coped with anti-gay bias will inevitably be part of the issues explored in a therapeutic process; many gay people–who have moved along the coming out process to self-acknowledgment–present themselves or express their sexual feelings to others with an expectation of being ignored or rejected. Such people will face the same fears in seeking help from medical or mental health providers, regardless of what the orientation of the provider may be. Treatment must focus on recovery from substance abuse and from the consequences of homophobia. To reverse and treat the denial and dissociation described above, the patient will need to address his or her own acceptance of self as a gay person. Although no one should be forced to come out to anyone, self-acceptance appears to be crucial to recovery. Treatment needs to be at least gay-sensitive if not gay-affirmative, as will be discussed below. To "recover" from the "Alice Miller"-type childhood, the patient, once in solid recovery, will need to address the grief and rage associated with mourning the loss of the "false self" and must learn how to get his or her own real needs met.

In the assessment of a gay man or lesbian presenting for mental health services, clinicians need to be aware of the higher incidence of substance abuse in this population and, accordingly, routinely screen for symptoms of alcoholism or other substance abuse. In formulating a treatment plan for gay men or lesbians determined to have a substance abuse problem, the assessment needs to explore the following for each individual: the stage in the life-cycle; the degree and impact of internalized homophobia; the stage in the coming-out process and the experience of coming out; the support and social network available; current relationship, if any, including married spouses and the history of past relationships; the relationship with the family of origin;

comfort with sexuality and expression of sexual feelings; career and economic status; and health factors, including HIV status.

Most clinicians working with the addictions recognize that exploratory psychotherapy alone will not treat or cure the substance abuse, and, in fact, may actually be harmful and not indicated (Vaillant, 1983). Traditional individual psychotherapy can be isolating and lonely, and may create the false hope that understanding and insight will lead to recovery; often, the insights lead to rationalizations for continuing to abuse substances. If a patient is already in therapy when recovery begins, the therapy need not stop, but the work will need to be much more supportive and focused on the here and now and the recovery process itself, while the emotional and neurological systems begin to heal. Once in solid recovery, the patient can deal with the grief and rage involved in mourning the loss of the "false self," the time lost living the false self, and learn how to get his or her own real needs met. A Twelve-Step program such as Alcoholics Anonymous (AA) is a vital part of recovery and is essential for all substance abusing patients who undertake psychotherapy.

Often, inpatient and outpatient detoxification and rehabilitation programs lack knowledge about homosexuality and are unaware that they have gay, lesbian, and bisexual patients, who may be too frightened to come out to the staff (Hellman et al., 1989). Many gay and lesbian staff are afraid to come out at work as well, because of administrative reaction and they are, therefore, not able to either serve as role models or provide a more open and relaxed treatment.

If treatment in a formal substance abuse program is indicated, the program should at least be gay-sensitive–aware of, knowledgeable about, and accepting of gay people in a non-prejudicial fashion. The ideal program would be gay-affirmative–actively promoting self-acceptance of a gay identity as a key part of recovery. With the greater awareness of the link between HIV infection and substance use and abuse, the treatment of substance abuse disorders is equivalent to HIV prevention.

Twelve-Step recovery programs and philosophies are the mainstays in staying free from drug use and alcohol use (living clean and sober) for most substance abusers. Many larger communities now have gay and lesbian AA, Narcotics Anonymous (NA), Cocaine Anonymous (CA), and Al-Anon meetings; AA, as an organization, clearly embraces gays and lesbians, as it embraces anyone concerned about a substance abuse problem (Kus, 1989). Some groups parallel and similar to AA have formed to meet the needs of gay men and lesbians, such as Alcoholics Together, and many big cities sponsor "round-ups"–large three day weekend gatherings focused on AA, NA, lectures, workshops, and drug- and alcohol-free socializing.

Though AA, CA, and NA recommend avoiding emotional stress and conflicts in the first six months of recovery, for the gay man or lesbian in such programs, relapse is almost certain if the gay person cannot acknowledge and accept his or her sexual orientation. Discussion of the conflicts about acknowledgment of sexual orientation and living comfortably as a gay person is essential for recovery, even if these topics are emotionally laden and stressful.

Many localities now have gay, lesbian, and bisexual health or mental health centers, almost all with a focus on recovery and substance abuse treatment. National organizations, such as the National Association of Lesbian and Gay Addiction Professionals, the Association of Gay and Lesbian Psychiatrists, the Gay and Lesbian Medical Association, the Association of Lesbian and Gay Psychologists, and the National Gay Social Workers, can help with appropriate referrals.

Some of the suggestions and guidelines of AA and NA and most treatment programs may be difficult for some gay men and lesbians to follow: giving up or avoiding old friends, especially fellow substance users, for the gay person if he or she has limited contacts who relate to him or her as a gay person; staying away from bars or parties if they are the only gay social outlets available. Special help on how to not drink or use drugs in such settings may be necessary. Many gay people mistakenly link AA and religion; because many religious institutions denounce or condemn homosexuality, gay men and lesbians may be resistant to trying AA or NA.

Other factors affect the treatment of gay men and lesbians. Many gay men and lesbians are in long-term relationships, and treatment for these individuals must clearly focus on relationships, parenting, and family concerns. Lesbians and gay men are also subject to an increase in violent attacks because of their sexual orientation, both verbal and physical (Klinger and Stein, 1996); reaction to such an attack may include relapse for a person already in recovery or an increase in use by someone currently using. In addition, many gay men and lesbians are victims of domestic violence. This latter fact is often ignored by clinicians; however, because there are correlations with domestic violence and substance abuse, clinicians need to be aware of this possible combination (Schilit, Lie, and Montagne,1990; Island and Letellier, 1991).

A brief list of additional treatment issues facing all people in recovery–with special impact on gays and lesbians–beyond the scope of this review includes: how to have safer sex while clean and sober; how to adjust to clean and sober socializing, without the use of alcohol or drugs to hide social anxiety; employment problems and adjustment to the impact of being out as a gay person at work; work with the family of origin regarding acceptance of the sexual orientation of their gay or lesbian child; couples adjusting to the damaging effects substance use may have had over the years; the negative impact of co-dependent relationships; confidentiality in record keeping, especially around discussion in the medical record of sexual orientation or HIV status; child custody issues when necessary; diagnosis and treatment of additional medical problems; and, legal problems. Finnegan and McNally (1987) address most of these concerns in greater detail.

ISSUES SPECIFIC FOR LESBIANS

As described above, the incidence of substance abuse is equally high for gay men and lesbians, but lesbians who abuse substances may have additional social struggles and concerns. Compared to gay men, lesbians are more likely to have lower incomes; lesbians are more likely to be parents–up to one-third of lesbians are biological parents (Kirkpatrick, 1996); lesbians face the prejudices aimed at women as well as those for being gay, including the stronger reaction against and willingness to ignore female substance abusers (Gartrell, 1983); lesbians are more likely to come out later in life (Herbert, 1996); and lesbians more often have bisexual feelings or experiences (Bell and Weinberg, 1978; Bell, Weinberg, and Hammersmith, 1981), and, as a result, are at greater risk for HIV-infection via a heterosexual sexual route in addition to possible IV-drug use and woman-to-woman transmission.

A few surveys have focused on lesbian substance abuse, one in the general population (Bradford and Ryan, 1987) and one in lesbian medical students (Mosbacher, 1993). Both continue to indicate a high use of alcohol and other drugs in lesbians, and a higher concern over a problem with alcohol and drug use than in similar heterosexual populations.

The following discussion looks at gay men more specifically. Some of the issues will also apply to lesbians but the factors involved in being "male" and "gay" in our society versus being "female" and "lesbian" lead to limited applications to lesbians for all the topics discussed below.

ISSUES SPECIFIC FOR GAY MEN

Being male brings its own social and cultural pressures in addition to those about being gay described above. Cultural expectations about what it means to be male, regardless of sexual orientation, add social and personal pressures. These cultural expectations–basically gender role expectations–vary by culture and ethnicity. Gay men of color may face quite different problems than those white gay men face.

In general though, a cultural stereotype of being male in America seems to be the expectation of being powerful, masculine, independent, emotionally reserved, career motivated rather than relationship motivated, and sexually driven with a focus on obtaining orgasm and having multiple partners. Boys and men who do not seem to fit this stereotype–or who do not wish to act like this stereotype–may have trouble fitting in or being comfortable with themselves.

Part of societal heterosexism stems from confusion about what homosexuality is and what gay men are. Since most heterosexuals cannot image what it is like to be gay, to be attracted to someone of the same sex, they often assume that a gay man must be in some way like a woman. If a man wants to be with another man emotionally or sexually, they think, then the gay man must see himself as a woman. Many cultures, especially Latin-based cultures, cast great stigma on any man who is like a woman. This stigma may be the basis for much of the anti-gay bias seen in America, and may be a major factor in homophobia.

Certainly some gay men may be "effeminate"–that is, they may have some traits that are culturally attributed to women. "Effeminacy" in and of itself has nothing to do with sexual orientation. Many "effeminate" men are heterosexual. Unless a gay man is also transgender, he does not think he is a woman or wish to be a woman.

Many gay men, though, do grow up different from their heterosexual peers, and a considerable percentage of gay boys and men may have traits and behaviors that are more associated with girls or women, such as avoidance of rough and tumble play, being less aggressive, or being less interested in sports. These traits do not cause homosexuality but they do predict a greater likelihood of homosexuality in adulthood. Such traits often lead to the child being stigmatized. Many gay men report feeling isolated, avoiding contact with the more "macho" types of guys in school–which of course adds to the stress of being different.

The prejudicial link between being gay and being effeminate or weak is sometimes believed even by gay men and generates more shame. Gay men who are more passive or who enjoy sex as the receiving partner may feel deep shame and embarrassment about that behavior and desire. That shame over being a "bottom," as defined by many gay men, may contribute to the use of drugs and alcohol.

Some gay men may feel pressure–even or especially by other gay men–to be more "butch," masculine behaving, or "macho" than they feel comfortable. This conflict may lead to acting more reserved or aloof in general, making it hard to be relaxed or feel themselves. This pressure to be a "top," as many gay men would describe the sexual insertor or aggressive role may also lead to drug and alcohol use, especially drugs that make one feel more sexual or enhance sexual performance such as amphetamines or amyl nitrate. The desire to be so masculine also contributes to the great focus on looks and body image for many gay men, including obsession with the body, working out, and use and abuse of steroids.

Types and Patterns of Substances Abused

Any and all types of drugs and alcohol may be used and abused by gay men or lesbians. There are however certain drugs used that may be more associated with this population–especially gay men–than others.

An explosive use of methamphetamine, known as "speed," "crystal," or "crank," by gay and bisexual men has become evident and of grave concern. There are many routes of administration, including oral inhalation, nasal insufflation, absorption through the rectal mucosa, and intravenous use. Combined with its effects of behavioral disinhibition and sexual stimulation, methamphetamine use puts some gay male users at extremely high risk for HIV infection (Gorman, Morgan, and Lambert, 1995).

"Circuit parties" are very popular with a segment of gay men and drug use is quite prominent and extensive in those settings. Drugs such as "Ecstasy," "Special K," gamma hydroxybutyrate (GHB), "Blue Nitro," and other "designer" drugs are very popular, in addition to alcohol, amphetamines, marijuana, and cocaine.

"Poppers" or inhaleable amyl nitrate or variants of it are also used by many people of all sexual orientations, but have been noted to play a significant role in sexual activity for many gay men. Again, not all gay men use these drugs or with these patterns, but certain drugs, such as amphetamines, are very difficult to stop using, and certain drugs associated with sexual behavior may be harder to give up than others.

Gay Male Social Life

Because gay men are so diverse, coming from every age group and ethnicity, there are no valid generalizations that can be made about gay men or even large segments of gay men. Urban life differs from suburban or rural life for gay men. Single gay men may live differently than men in relationships; younger gay men differently than older men; men of color differently than white men. Obviously such diversity cannot be squeezed into stereotypes.

The popular media portrays gay men in various stereotypes such as young, beautiful, materialistic, and focused on sex and partying; or, older, strange looking, into leather and kinky things; or, into drag (dressing up as women) and/or acting quite effeminate. Of course there are gay men who will fit each of those stereotypes, but most do not fit into any of these groups.

Many young gay men, just coming out, with limited or no role models, may believe these indeed are the ways one has to be. Many gay men of all ages will see pressure to somehow be like the "gay man" they see in the popular gay press or the general media–young, thin, well-built, usually white, and sexually focused–and feel that there is "ageism," "looksism," and even racism in the "gay community." Again, these "isms" may exist in certain individuals but they cannot be attributed to all gay men.

Gay men of color sometimes describe feeling invisible in settings where most of the other gay men are white, though this experience varies by city, location, and region of the country. In addition, they may have specific cultural or ethnic issues about homosexuality or ways of having sex, as may many white gay men. For example, many cultures may not condem sex between men but at the same time condemn or ridicule a man who takes the receptive role in sex. A man can have sex with another man–but not really talk about it–if he is the active or insertive partner, especially if he is married to a woman or considers himself straight (or at most bisexual) even if he mainly has sex with other men.

In spite of more awareness and acceptance of gay people, gay social outlets still tend to be limited both in scope and location. The "gay ghetto" is the section of town where gay people feel comfortable in hanging out and getting together–usually marked by gay bars. Though there are more gay coffee shops and bookstores and non-alcohol and drug-related locations and activities, bars and parties that focus on alcohol and drug use are the best advertised and easily identified parts of gay social life.

An activity that seems unique to gay people–mostly men though some lesbians take part–are weekend long gatherings that focus on dancing, partying, sexual activity, and drug and alcohol use called "circuit parties." These parties, attended primarily by gay men in their early 20's to late 40's, are held all around the world, forming a "circuit" of connected activities and frequented by many of the same people who go from event to event. The parties encourage drug use–to enhance the dancing (a "rave") and to enhance sexual activity. "Designer" drugs such as Ecstasy, GHB, Special-K, amphetamines, and others are heavily used and promoted. There have even been fatalities associated with the use of drugs at some of these parties.

Sexual Activity

Just as in almost all parts of our society, there is a strong emphasis on sex in the media targeted to gay men. Many people think of gay men as sexually obsessed, as a result of the general media's focus on gay male sexual activity especially when looking at HIV and AIDS. Gay men are probably no more sexually obsessed or active than men in general.

There is a small subsection of gay men who are focused on sexual activity with many partners and/or with great frequency. Many of these men have discovered cocaine and amphetamine use to be a great enhancer of sexual intensity and activity. Amphetamines in particular seem to increase and prolong sexual feelings and sexual stamina. Many gay men who use amphetamines also develop a side effect associated with amphetamines–transient impotence. Sexual desire is still greatly enhanced–for up to 14 hours–and these men will be anal-receptive partners, sometimes with many partners, and are at greater risk for HIV infection if precautions are not followed.

Another social outlet mostly associated with gay men (though again lesbians as well as some heterosexual people have such outlets) are sex clubs and bathhouses or private gyms with areas for sexual activity. For many gay men, still uncomfortable with going to gay activities or bars, or who do not wish to be in a steady relationship, or who want sexual adventure, these venues are popular and exciting. The vast majority of these types of places ban the use of drugs or alcohol, but these rules are variably enforced and many gay men–strongly linking sexual activity with drug or alcohol use–will get "high" before going to the location.

Gay Male Life Cycles and Relationships

Gay men at each stage of their lives may face challenges unique to being gay. Adolescents who are gay or bisexual or questioning if they are gay or bisexual, for example, face possible taunts or threats from their peers. Their families may reject them and some gay youth run away from home. These young men may end up homeless and may also get into drug use (especially IV use) and turn to prostitution. This author has consulted with several gay youth who were living on the street and reported attempting to acquire an HIV infection so that they would qualify for medical and social services as well as disability incomes and housing programs!

The suicide risk may be three times that of other youth, including ideation, attempts, and completed suicides (Rotheram-Borus, Hunter, and Rosario, 1994). Gay youth also face more problems with schoolwork, sexual abuse, and drug and alcohol use even if they do not leave home. The experimentation with drugs and sex will certainly be part of the development of gay youth even if accepted by family and self-accepting–just as with any adolescent or young adult.

Most gay men form relationships but same-sex relationships are not readily accepted or even acknowledged in America (Cabaj, 1988; Cabaj and Purcell, 1998). Gay people are still fighting for the right for same-sex marriage. Many gay men have children–either by a marriage or relationship with a woman, by adoption, or by a co-parenting relationship with a lesbian friend, for example–and face the struggles of raising children with little support from society or even from other gay people. Such pressures may contribute to drug and alcohol use.

Older gay men face the same issues as all older people but may feel more isolated and disconnected from others because of having grown up gay at a time of even greater prejudice and denial of gay people. Many gay men, though, have developed strengths from years of battling anti-gay bias that serve them well in coping with aging. Some older men will be facing the loss of a long term relationship; such "gay widows" may have few social supports. Of course, drug and alcohol use may be a major part of an older gay man's life and will need interventions that address both the concerns of aging and being gay.

CONCLUSIONS

Traditional psychotherapy with an active substance abuser is usually contraindicated. Supportive, motivational therapy may help the person to recognize the need to address the substance use, and can serve as a bridge into addiction treatment. Psychotherapy can begin in the early recovery period, or–if the patient was a substance abuser but not addicted and has been able to reduce or eliminate the drug or alcohol use–at the point the patient can discuss honestly the use and the effect on his or her life.

The description of gay men's and lesbians' lives affected by parents who could not acknowledge or accept the true selves of those individuals applies to many but not all gay men and lesbians. Substance using and abusing gay people, though, will have some defense mechanisms that may be a result of chronic drug or alcohol use, such as denial, projection, and distortion, and these defenses may be compounded by developmental issues.

The many issues discussed above will help frame the best approach to the individual gay man or lesbian who is abusing drugs or alcohol. Ongoing psychotherapy, whether it is exploratory, supportive, cognitive behavioral, or group, will need to be done with the awareness that relapse is frequent in the addicted patient and that life stressors may lead to increased use in the abusing patient. Each relapse can be a learning process–exploring what led to the relapse and how to avoid it in the future. Psychotherapy during a relapse is then quite difficult, if not impossible, to do–it will inevitably take on a supportive nature–but recovery or reduced use is always the goal and will then allow further exploration in psychotherapy.

REFERENCES

Bailey, J. M. & Benishay, D. S. (1993), Familial aggregation of female sexual orientation. *Amer. J. Psychiat.* 150(2):272-277.

_____ & Pillard, R. C. (1991), A genetic study of male sexual orientation. *Arch. Gen. Psychiat.* 48:1089-1096.

Beatty, R. (1983), Alcoholism and adult gay male populations of Pennsylvania. Unpublished master's thesis, Pennsylvania State University.

Bell, A. P. & Weinberg, M. S. (1978), *Homosexualities: A Study of Diversities Among Men and Women.* New York: Simon and Schuster.

_____, _____ & Hammersmith, S. K. (1981), *Sexual Preference: Its Development in Men and Women.* Bloomington, IN: Indiana University Press.

Bradford, J. & Ryan, C. (1987), Mental health implications: National lesbian health care survey. Unpublished report for the National Lesbian and Gay Health Foundation, Washington, DC.

Cabaj, R. P. (1988), Gay and lesbian couples: Lessons on human intimacy. *Psychiat. Annals.* 18(1), 21-25.

_____ (1997), Gays, lesbians, and bisexuals. In: *Substance Abuse: A Comprehensive Textbook, Third Edition,* ed. J. H. Lowenson, P. Ruiz, R. P. Millman & J. G. Langrod. Baltimore: Williams and Wilkins, pp. 725-733.

_____ (1985), Homophobia: A hidden factor in psychotherapy. *Contemporary Psychiat.* 4(3):135-137.

_____ & Purcell, D.W., ed. (1998), *On the Road to Same-Sex Marriage: A Supportive Guide to Psychological, Political, and Legal Issues*. San Francisco, CA: Jossey-Bass Publishers.

Cass, V. (1996), Sexual orientation identity formation: A Western phenomenon. In: *Textbook of Homosexuality and Mental Health*, ed. R. P. Cabaj & T. S. Stein. Washington, DC: American Psychiatric Press, Inc., pp. 227-251.

Cassel, J. (1976), The contributions of the social environment to host resistance. *Amer. J. Epidemiology*. 104:107-123.

Centers for Disease Control and Prevention. (1998), *HIV/AIDS Surveillance Report*. 10(2), 1-43.

Coleman, E. (1982), Developmental stages in the coming out process. *J. Homosexuality*. 7:31-43.

De Cecco, J. P., ed. (1984), *Homophobia: An Overview*. New York: The Haworth Press, Inc.

de Monteflores, C. (1996), Notes on the management of difference. In: *Contemporary Perspectives on Psychotherapy with Lesbians and Gay Men*, ed. T. S. Stein & C. C. Cohen. New York: Plenum, pp. 73-101.

_____ & Schultz, S. J. (1978), Coming out: Similarities and differences for lesbians and gay men. *J. Social Issues*. 34:59-73.

Diamond, D. L. & Wilsnack, S. C. (1978), Alcohol abuse among lesbians: A descriptive study. *J. Homosexuality*. 4(2):123-142.

Fifield, L., de Crescenzo, T. A. & Latham, J. D. (1975), On my way to nowhere: Alienated, isolated, drunk: An analysis of gay alcohol abuse and evaluation of alcoholism rehabilitation services for Los Angeles County. Unpublished report for Los Angeles Gay Community Services Center.

Finnegan, D. G. & McNally, E. B. (1987), *Dual Identities: Counseling Chemically Dependent Gay Men and Lesbians*. Center City, MN: Hazelden.

Forstein, M. (1988), Homophobia: An overview. *Psychiat. Annals*. 18(1):33-36.

Gartrell, N. (1983), Gay patients in the medical setting. In: *Treatment Interventions in Human Sexuality*, ed. C. Nadelson & D. Marcotte. New York: Plenum Press.

Gorman, E. M., Morgan, P. & Lambert, E.Y. (1995), Qualitative research considerations and other issues in the study of methamphetamine use among men who have sex with other men. In: *Qualitative Methods in Drug Abuse and HIV Research*, ed. R. Needle & E. Y. Lambert. Washington, DC: NIDA Research Monograph Series.

Hanley-Hackenbruck, P. (1988), "Coming-out" and psychotherapy. *Psychiat. Annals*. 18(1):29-32.

Hanson, G. & Hartmann, L. (1996), Latency development in prehomosexual boys. In: *Textbook of Homosexuality and Mental Health*, ed. R. P. Cabaj & T. S. Stein. Washington, DC: American Psychiatric Press, Inc., pp. 253-266.

Hellman, R. E., Stanton, M., Lee, J., Tytun, A. & Vachon, R. Treatment of homosexual alcoholics in government-funded agencies: Provider training and attitudes. *Hosp. Community Psychiat*. 40(11):1163-1168.

Herbert, S. E. (1996), Lesbian sexuality. In: *Textbook of Homosexuality and Mental Health*, ed. R. P. Cabaj & T. S. Stein. Washington, DC: American Psychiatric Press, Inc., pp. 723-742.

Herek, G. M. (1996), Heterosexism and homophobia. In: *Textbook of Homosexuality and Mental Health*, ed. R. P. Cabaj & T. S. Stein. Washington, DC: American Psychiatric Press, Inc., pp. 65-82.

Hetrick, E. S. & Martin, A. D. (1987), Developmental issues and their resolution for gay and lesbian adolescents. *J. Homosexuality.* 14(1/2):25-44.

Isay, R. A. (1989), *Being Homosexual: Gay Men and Their Development.* New York: Farrar, Straus & Giroux.

Island, D. & Letellier, P. (1991), *Men Who Beat the Men Who Love Them: Battered Gay Men and Domestic Violence.* New York: Harrington Park Press.

Israelstam, S. & Lambert, S. (1983), Homosexuality as a cause of alcoholism: A historical review. *Internat. J. Addictions.* 18(8):1085-1107.

_____ (1986), Homosexuality and alcohol: Observations and research after the psychoanalytic era. *Internat. J. Addictions.* 21(4-5):509-537.

_____ (1989), Homosexuals who indulge in excessive use of alcohol and drugs: Psychosocial factors to be taken into account by community and intervention workers. *J. Alcohol and Drug Education.* 34(3):54-69.

Kirkpatrick, M. (1996), Lesbians as parents. In: *Textbook of Homosexuality and Mental Health*, ed. R. P. Cabaj & T. S. Stein. Washington, DC: American Psychiatric Press, Inc., pp. 353-370.

Klinger, R. L. & Stein, T. S. (1996), Impact of violence, childhood sexual abuse, and domestic violence and abuse on lesbian, bisexual, and gay men. In: *Textbook of Homosexuality and Mental Health*, ed. R. P. Cabaj & T. S. Stein. Washington, DC: American Psychiatric Press, Inc., pp. 801-818.

Kus, R. J. (1987), Alcoholics Anonymous and gay American men. *J. Homosexuality.* 14 (1/2):253-276.

Lesbian and Gay Substance Abuse Planning Group. (1991), San Francisco Lesbian, Gay and Bisexual Substance Abuse Needs Assessment. Unpublished report.

Lewis, C. E., Saghir, M. T. & Robins, E. (1982), Drinking patterns in homosexual and heterosexual women. *J. Clin. Psychiat.* 43:277-279.

Lohrenz, L., Connelly, J., Coyne, L. & Spare, K. (1987), Alcohol problems in several midwestern homosexual communities. *J. Studies on Alcohol.* 39(11):1959-1963.

Martin, A. D. (1982), Learning to hide: The socialization of the gay adolescent. *Adolescent Psychiat.* 10:52-65.

McDonald, G. (1982), Individual differences in the coming out process for gay men: Implications for theoretical models. *J. Homosexuality.* 8:47-60.

McKirnan, D. & Peterson, P. L. (1989a), Alcohol and drug abuse among homosexual men and women: Epidemiology and population characteristics. *Addictive Behaviors.* 14:545-553.

_____ (1989b), Psychological and cultural factors in alcohol and drug abuse: An analysis of a homosexual community. *Addictive Behaviors.* 14:555-563.

Miller, A. (1981), *The Drama of the Gifted Child.* New York: Basic Books.

_____ (1984), *For Your Own Good: Hidden Cruelty in Child-rearing and the Roots of Violence.* New York: Farrar, Straus, & Giroux.

Morales, E. S. & Graves, M. A. (1983), Substance Abuse: Patterns and Barriers to Treatment for Gay Men and Lesbians in San Francisco. Unpublished report for San Francisco Prevention Resources Center.

Mosbacher, D. (1988), Lesbian alcohol and substance abuse. *Psychiat. Annals.* 18(1):47-50.

_____ (1993), Alcohol and other drug use in female medical students: A comparison of lesbians and heterosexuals. *J. Gay & Lesbian Psychotherapy.* 2(1):37-48.

Pillard, R. C. (1988), Sexual orientation and mental disorder. *Psychiat. Annals.* 18(1):52-56.

_____ , Poumadere, J. & Carretta, R. A. (1982), A family study of sexual orientation. *Arch. Sexual Behavior.* 11(6):511-520.

_____ & Weinrich, J. D. (1986), Evidence of familial nature of male sexuality. *Arch. Gen. Psychiat.* 43:808-812.

Rotheram-Borus, M. J., Hunter, J. & Rosario, M. (1994), Suicidal behavior and gay-related stress among gay and bisexual male adolescents. *J. Adolescent Research.* 9:498-508.

Saghir, M. & Robins, E. (1973), *Male and Female Homosexuality.* Baltimore: Williams and Wilkins.

Schilit, R., Lie, G. Y. & Montagne, M. (1990), Substance use as a correlate of violence in intimate lesbian relationships. *J. Homosexuality.* 19(3):51-65.

Stall, R. & Wiley, J. (1988), A comparison of alcohol and drug use patterns of homosexual and heterosexual men: The San Francisco Men's Health Study. *Drug and Alcohol Dependency.* 22:63-73.

Vaillant, G. E. (1983), *The Natural History of Alcoholism: Causes, Patterns, and Paths to Recovery.* Cambridge, MA: Harvard University Press.

Weinberg, G. (1972), *Society and the Healthy Homosexual.* New York: St. Martin's Press.

Weinberg, M. & Williams, C. (1974), *Male Homosexuals: Their Problems and Adaptations.* New York: Oxford University Press.

The Prevalence of Alcoholism
and Feelings of Alienation
in Lesbian and Heterosexual Women

Carrie Jaffe, PhD
Pauline Rose Clance, PhD
Margaret F. Nichols, PhD
James G. Emshoff, PhD

SUMMARY. Although only a handful of studies have examined alcoholism among lesbians, high rates of alcoholism among lesbians are often reported. This study investigated the prevalence of alcoholism and its relation to feelings of alienation in samples of lesbian and heterosexual women. It was hypothesized that alienation would correlate with alcoholism. The sample consisted of 87 lesbian and 89 heterosexual women obtained from women's groups. Questionnaires included the Michigan Alcoholism Screening Test, the Dean Alienation Scale, and the Kinsey Rating Scale. Significant differences were found between lesbian and heterosexual women on alcoholism and on the Powerlessness subscale of the Dean. Alienation did not correlate with alcoholism in the lesbian sample. *[Article copies available for a fee from The Haworth Document Delivery Service: 1-800-342-9678. E-mail address: <getinfo@haworth pressinc.com> Website: <http://www.HaworthPress.com>]*

Dr. Carrie Jaffe is a director of a drug and alcohol prevention and treatment program for youths in Hayward, CA. Dr. Pauline Rose Clance is Professor of Psychology, Georgia State University. Dr. Margaret F. Nichols is Adjunct Professor of Psychology, Georgia State University and has a private practice in Atlanta. Dr. James G. Emshoff is Professor of Community Psychology, Georgia State University.

Address correspondence to: Dr. Carrie Jaffe, Dr. Pauline Rose Clance, and Dr. James G. Emshoff, all at the Psychology Department, Georgia State University, University Plaza, Atlanta, GA 30303. Dr. Margaret F. Nichols can be reached at 1293 Peachtree Street, Suite 730, Atlanta, GA 30309.

[Haworth co-indexing entry note]: "The Prevalence of Alcoholism and Feelings of Alienation in Lesbian and Heterosexual Women." Jaffe, Carrie et al. Co-published simultaneously in *Journal of Gay & Lesbian Psychotherapy* (The Haworth Medical Press, an imprint of The Haworth Press, Inc.) Vol. 3, No. 3/4, 2000, pp. 25-35; and: *Addictions in the Gay and Lesbian Community* (ed: Jeffrey R. Guss, and Jack Drescher) The Haworth Medical Press, an imprint of The Haworth Press, Inc., 2000, pp. 25-35. Single or multiple copies of this article are available from The Haworth Document Delivery Service [1-800-342-9678, 9:00 a.m. - 5:00 p.m. (EST). E-mail address: getinfo@haworthpressinc.com].

© 2000 by The Haworth Press, Inc. All rights reserved.

KEYWORDS. Alcoholism, lesbian, alienation, powerlessness, Michigan Alcoholism Screening Test, Dean Alienation Scale

Recently, there has been an increase in the attention paid to drinking patterns and the rate of alcoholism in the lesbian community. Statements can easily be found in the psychological literature that are suggestive of alcohol problems in the lesbian community (Saghir, Robins, Walbran, & Gentry, 1970; Fifield, Latham, & Phillips, 1977; Lewis, Saghir, & Robins, 1982). For example, Nicoloff and Stiglitz (1987) asserted, "alcohol abuse and alcoholism are significant problems for the lesbian population; [they] appear to be more severe for lesbians than for heterosexual women or for the heterosexual community at large." McKirnan and Peterson (1989) noted, "homosexuals are substantially more likely than the general population to have an alcohol or drug problem." Finally, Zehner and Lewis (1984) stated, "among the gay and lesbian population, probably 20%-30% are alcoholic, twice to three times as large a percentage as in the general population" (p. 75).

However, a recurrent problem in the field of research with lesbians and gays is a habitual paucity of literature. In 1982, Nardi found only 42 references listed under homosexuality in the index of the *Journal of Studies on Alcohol,* a primary publication in the field of alcoholism. Only 10 of those 42 directly examined alcohol use by lesbians and gay men. The remainder consisted of psychoanalytic research and studies which utilized sexual preference for demographic data only. Four years after Nardi's review, in 1986, Israelstam and Lambert found 32 articles in their review of the literature on alcoholism and gays. Our own review of the literature revealed an additional 10 articles, resulting in a grand total of 42 (the same number found by Nardi in 1982). As has been the case with heterosexual women in substance abuse studies, lesbians have typically been studied as a part of larger groups of gay men. Findings from these studies are expected to generalize to both women and men, although the overwhelming majority of these groups is male.

In 1988, Mosbacher found only five studies that examined lesbian alcoholism. Two focused solely on lesbians while three others included lesbians only as part of another population. Mosbacher noted some methodological limitations of these studies, including small sample sizes, a lack of operational definitions (often absent in studies which measure alcohol problems and alcoholism and categorize women as lesbian), and the use of instruments which do not demonstrate adequate validity or reliability.

Recently, several studies have emerged, in which the authors, in addition to investigating rates of alcoholism, examined social and political alienation and internalized homophobia as possible reasons lesbians often turn to alcohol. Schilit, Lie, and Montagne (1990) stated, "alienation, isolation, and oppression are facts of life for lesbians in this country. Many lesbians are finding an escape with alcohol . . . " Glaus (1989) theorized that internalized homophobia, or the internalization of societal homophobia creates internal conflict for lesbians that can lead to high rates of alcohol use. Saunders and Valente (1987) stated gays and lesbians experience alienation from society due to societal homophobia. They further stated alienation in gay men and lesbians is likely to continue as long as they are denied equal rights and privileges of larger society.

LITERATURE REVIEW

Saghir, Robins, Walbran, and Gentry (1970) examined psychiatric disorders in lesbians. Fifty-seven lesbian women, obtained from lesbian organizations, and 43 single heterosexuals obtained from an apartment complex and "word of mouth" were interviewed to determine and compare the degree of psychiatric disorder and disability in these two groups. The criterion for defining sexual orientation was exclusive sexual behavior with one gender or the other after the age of 18. All subjects were Caucasian. Results indicated 10% (6) of the lesbian subjects were alcohol dependent, compared to none of the heterosexual subjects; an additional 25% (14) lesbian women were found to drink excessively, compared to 5% (2) of the controls. The 35% figure of alcohol problems exhibited in the lesbian women was considered the prevalent finding of this study.

Bradford and Ryan (1987) investigated the amount and frequency of alcohol use of 1971 lesbians as part of the National Lesbian Health Care Survey, a large study concerning general health care issues for lesbians. Questions concerning amount and frequency of alcohol use were included as part of a comprehensive health survey that was distributed to lesbians in major metropolitan cities throughout the United States. Results indicated approximately one-third of the sample used alcohol regularly, and 14% of the sample reported feeling worried about their alcohol use. Specifically, 6% of the sample drank daily, 25% drank weekly, 30% drank monthly, and 17% abstained.

McKirnan and Peterson (1989) distributed questionnaires to 3400 lesbians and gays, 22% of whom were lesbian. Twenty-three percent of the lesbian sample reported alcohol problems, compared to 8% of the general population.[1]

Lewis, Saghir, and Robins (1982) did the only investigation that focused solely on the comparison of lesbian women with heterosexual women on problem drinking. They utilized a structured interview that queried sexual orientation, drinking history, familial alcoholism, and frequency of gay bar attendance. The criterion for inclusion as a lesbian subject was a self-reported history of lesbian orientation and overt same sex behavior past age 18. The instrument used to assess alcoholism was a modification of a questionnaire used in a previous study by Guze (1976), an instrument that lacks validity and reliability data. The sample consisted of 43 Caucasian heterosexual women, obtained from an apartment complex, and 57 Caucasian lesbian women who were obtained from a national lesbian organization, referrals from previous subjects, and gay bars.

Results were three fold: 33% of the lesbian women reported heavy drinking or questionable alcoholism compared to 7% of the heterosexuals; 28% of the lesbian women were found to be alcoholic, compared with 5% of the heterosexuals, and; overall, lesbian subjects had a significantly higher rate of alcohol consumption than heterosexuals. Unfortunately, however, this study's generalizability is questionable due to its small, all white sample, its lack of operational definitions, and its use of instruments that lack validity and reliability data.

The purpose of the current study is to conceptually replicate important aspects of the Lewis, Saghir, and Robins (1982) study, while instituting fundamental changes. Conceptually, the Lewis et al. study is a good one, but it has problems in several essential areas. First, the Lewis et al. study lacks a large and broad enough subject population. Thus it is generalizable only to its three subject sources and only to white women who are without any serious clinical or legal histories (which many alcoholics are prone to have). Second, no reliability or validity data are available for the instruments used in Lewis et al. Finally, clear operationally defined constructs were not used in Lewis et al. to define sexual orientation. This study is an attempt to improve on the above three weaknesses of the original study by using operationally defined constructs, reliable and valid instruments, and a broad sample size.

There were two hypotheses: (a) the prevalence of alcoholism among the lesbian subject sample would be higher than among the heterosexual sample, and (b) societal alienation would correlate with alcoholism in the lesbian sample.

METHOD

Subjects were 87 lesbian and 89 heterosexual women obtained through local women's associations, such as professional groups, religious groups, and bookstores. Wherever possible, equal numbers of heterosexual and lesbian women were obtained from comparable settings. In situations where this was not possible, as in cases of exclusively lesbian groups, data were obtained from matched heterosexual groups. Groups were matched based on their purpose and socioeconomic status of the members.

Sexual orientation was defined with a modified version of the Kinsey Rating Scale (Kinsey, Pomeroy, and Martin, 1953), a self report instrument which measures overt sexual behavior for the preceding two years. Lesbians were defined as women who had sexual relationships exclusively with women for at least the past two years. Heterosexuals were defined as women who had sexual relationships exclusively with men for at least the past two years. Bisexuals were not included in the study.

Subjects were also given the Michigan Alcoholism Screening Test

(MAST, Selzer, 1971), the Dean Alienation Scale (Dean, 1961), and a questionnaire gathering demographic information. Instruments were paper and pencil measures that were completed by the subjects; they were given in person by the experimenter. These measures are described below.

Instruments

Michigan Alcoholism Screening Test (MAST). The MAST is a self-report instrument, which screens for alcoholism. It consists of 25 true/false questions, which measure frequency, pattern, and consequences of drinking. Alcoholism is defined as a score of five or higher. Skinner and Sheu (1982) found reliability for the MAST to be high, at .84. Mischke and Venneri (1987) demonstrated internal consistency reliability, and Zung and Charalampous (1975) found the MAST to be valid in a sample of DWI offenders.

Due to its sensitivity, the MAST is more likely to result in overreporting rather than underreporting of alcoholism (Moore, 1972). Moore stated that, because the MAST is a screening instrument, rather than a diagnostic tool, overreporting is preferable to underreporting. This sensitivity is also viewed as a strength in the present study.

Dean Alienation Scale. The scale is divided into three subscales: Powerlessness, which relates to feelings of helplessness in the areas of one's economic destiny and influence over the course of public and political events; Normlessness, which relates to an uneasy or anxious "feeling of separation from group status" (Dean, 1961; p. 754) and a feeling of loss of direction in one's life; and Social Isolation, which is related to a feeling of "isolation from group standards" (Dean, p. 755). It is a Likert-type scale with a total of 24 questions. According to Dean, reliability coefficients for the three subscales are .78, .73, and .84, respectively. The total Alienation Score has a reliability coefficient of .78.

RESULTS

A multivariate analysis of variance (MANOVA) was performed to test for differences between groups of lesbian and heterosexual women on mean scores for the MAST and the Dean Alienation Scale.

Table 1 presents the means and standard deviations for MAST and Dean Alienation Scale scores for lesbian and heterosexual women. The MANOVA indicated significant differences between groups. Analyses showed that lesbian women reported higher levels of alcoholism than heterosexual women, $F(1, 176) = 5.11$, ($p < .05$). A significant difference was also found on the Dean Powerlessness subscale. Heterosexual women scored significantly higher than lesbians on this scale, $F(2,176) = 4.62$, $p < .05$. No differences were found on the Normlessness or Social Isolation subscales, or the total Alienation score.

TABLE 1. Descriptive Statistics for Major Variables

Lesbian/Heterosexual Women

Variable	Mean	Standard Deviation	Minimum	Maximum
MAST	7.76/4.29	11.38/8.84	0/0	51/49
Dean Alienation Scale				
Total Score	63.31/66.2	11.18/10.67	38/38	101/91
Normlessness	14.36/15.18	3.58/3.71	6/6	22/23
Isolation	23.07/22.83	7.54/4.69	12/10	77/36
Powerlessness	26.58/28.18	5.00/4.91	16/16	43/38

Chi-square analyses were performed to determine whether there was a relationship between sexual orientation and demographic characteristics (see Table 2). Age, educational status, personal and family income, and type of employment were tested. The lesbian and heterosexual samples were distributed equally across age and personal and family income, while significant differences were found for educational status and type of employment. Twenty-two percent of the lesbian sample had either a Master's degree, PhD, or MD, compared to 9% of the heterosexual sample (X^2 (7, 176) = 18.88, $p <$ .001). Forty-three percent of the lesbian sample held professional, managerial or technical jobs compared to 32% of the heterosexual sample, while 17% of the heterosexual sample held trade-related, clerical, or service positions, compared to 7% of the lesbian sample (X^2(4, 176) = 13.93, $p < .01$).

Chi-square analysis was also performed on all relationship variables. Relationship variables included whether the subject was in a relationship, and if so, the status of the relationship as monogamous or non-monogamous, the length of the relationship, the presence of a formal commitment in the relationship, cohabitation status, and whether the couple was married or dating (Table 3). The two groups were found to be distributed equally across relationship variables, with the exception of marital status. Four percent of the lesbian sample described their relational status as "married," while 48% of the heterosexual sample were married.

To investigate the interrelationships among measures, pearson product moment correlations were computed for all pairs of variables. As shown in Table 4, none of the correlations was statistically significant.

DISCUSSION

Lesbian subjects in this sample had a significantly higher prevalence of alcoholism than did a matched cohort of heterosexual women, as predicted. Eighteen percent of the lesbian sample scored six or higher on the MAST

TABLE 2. Demographic Variables

Variable	Means Lesbian	Means Heterosexual	Total
Age	32	36	34
Personal Income	$28,000	$22,000	$25,000
Family Income	$35,000	$37,000	$36,000
		Percents	
Race			
Caucasian	–	–	95%
African American	–	–	3%
Native American	–	–	1%
Asian or Hispanic	–	–	1%
Educational Status			
College Completion	38%	46%	94%
Professional Degree	22%	9%	31%
Type of Employment			
Professional, Managerial,			
Technical	43%	32%	75%
Trade, Clerical, or Service	17%	7%	24%

TABLE 3. Distribution of Subjects Across Relationship Variables

	% Lesbian	Heterosexual
Monogamous	96%	98%
Non-Monogamous	4%	2%
Committed		
Relationship	51%	42%
Non-Committed		
Relationship	8%	10%
Dating	6%	13%
No Relationship	35%	35%
Living Together	32%	18%
Married	4%	48%

compared to 7% of heterosexual subjects, demonstrating higher levels of alcoholism. This is consistent with previous findings, although the prevalence of alcoholism among lesbians is slightly higher in this study. One possible reason for this is the MAST, as a screening instrument, is likely to overreport rather than underreport alcoholism (Moore, 1972). Therefore, higher rates are expected with the MAST than with diagnostic interview

TABLE 4. Correlational Matrix of Variables

	MAST	Normlessness	Isolation	Powerlessness	Total
Length	−.14*	−.05	−.10	−.00	−.05
MAST		.02	.06	−.05	−.00
Normlessness			.36**	.59**	.81**
Isolation				.37**	.59**
Powerlessness					.85**

*$p < .05$ **$p < .001$

assessments reported in other studies (e.g., Lewis, Saghir, & Robins, 1982; McKirnan & Peterson, 1989; Bradford & Ryan, 1987).

Our hypothesis that a higher level of alcoholism in lesbian women could be accounted for by feelings of alienation was not supported, as groups did not differ in alienation, nor did alienation correlate with alcoholism. Although it cannot be concluded from this research that higher levels of alcoholism are due to feelings of societal alienation in lesbians, higher levels of alcoholism in the gay community may be attributed to societal oppression and internalized homophobia. This possibility has been noted in other studies (Glaus, 1989; Schilit, Lie, & Montagne, 1990), as well as in Fifield et al. (1977) and Lohrenz, Connelly, Coyne, and Spare (1978) who examined alcoholism in gay males.

The type of societal alienation experienced by lesbians may be different from that which was measured in this study. The alienation scale used here measures hopelessness and powerlessness, but because of the recent gain in political power seen by lesbians and gay men, lesbians may not feel hopeless and powerless in society. Rather, their alienation may be experienced as an internalization of society's homophobia. It is possible that a measure of stress or internalized homophobia may prove fruitful in future studies.

This hypothesis is supported by arguments made by Saunders and Valente (1987), who stated that gays experience alienation in society due to their limited access to societal privileges because of discrimination against them which, in this country is legal. They further stated that groups who have been cut off from larger society in this way decrease alienation by banding together into close communities with shared norms and values. An alternative society is, therefore, formed which acts to reduce the alienation and powerlessness within that group.

Heterosexual women were found to experience feelings of powerlessness significantly more frequently than lesbian women. It is likely that women (the heterosexual sample, in this case) with lower levels of personal income, education, and employment would be more likely to experience feelings of powerlessness than women (the lesbian sample) with higher levels of personal income, education, and employment, as these are greatly valued in society. Higher income, education level, and employment status likely correspond with feelings of powerfulness in women.

This study illustrates several issues of consequence for therapists to bear in mind when providing mental health services to lesbians. First and foremost, because alcoholism rates are high in the lesbian community, it is important to take a thorough history of the lesbian client's alcohol use, regardless of the presenting problem. Second, although it was not tested in this study, several authors have focused on the issue of internalized homophobia, stress, and/or alienation among lesbians, which is likely to be a contributing factor to alcoholism or other symptoms of inner conflict. It is important that therapists who work with lesbians attend to these issues within the context of any presenting problem.

Of equal importance is the need for addiction and substance abuse treatment services specifically designed for lesbians. The etiology of alcoholism among lesbians is as yet unknown. However, the fact that alcoholism has been found to be more prevalent for lesbians than heterosexual women is evidence that addiction services need to be tailored to the special needs of lesbians. These special needs include a safe place to be "out" without being stigmatized or subject to other forms of homophobia. On the other hand, if a lesbian is more comfortable not disclosing her emotional and sexual orientation, this decision must be respected. Addiction programs that include family treatment as a part of the program must be supportive of significant others, whether they include lovers or friends. Finally, because little is known about the etiology of alcoholism in lesbians, a stance of open acceptance is encouraged concerning individual factors in the client's life that may be related to alcohol abuse or dependence.

An interesting finding in the present study was that groups were similar in terms of relationship variables. It is frequently believed that gay relationships are less monogamous and committed than those of heterosexual relationships, but subjects in this sample were involved in relationships which were relatively similar on those variables. The only difference, a significant one, was that of marital status, an obvious difference due to legal sanctions against lesbian marriages. For this reason, many lesbian couples who describe themselves as monogamous do not describe themselves as married. Even though such a large difference exists on this variable, the difference seems to be one of labelling, not relationships, per se. Groups were equally distributed across variables of monogamy, length of relationship, and level of commitment.

As is common in most research with gays, this study is limited by sample bias, as all women were obtained through organized groups, resulting in the exclusion of lesbians who are either not out, or choose not to participate in the lesbian community. Although an effort was made to reach all socioeconomic groups, the majority of subjects who participated in this inquiry were from well-educated and professional backgrounds. Minority women were also underrepresented in this study. Further research is needed with a greater diversity of samples. In light of its limitations, our results provide further evidence of alcohol abuse and dependence as an important mental health issue for lesbians.

NOTE

1. General population data are based on an earlier study by Clark and Midanik (19), in which the epidemiology of alcoholism was measured in a general population sample.

REFERENCES

Bradford, J., & Ryan, C. (1987), National lesbian health care survey mental health implications. Washington DC: National Lesbian and Gay Health Foundation. (NTIS No. PB88-201496).

Dean, D. (1961), Alienation: its meaning and measurement. *American Sociological Review*, 26: 753-758.

Diamond, D., & Wilsnack, S. (1978), Alcohol abuse among lesbians: a descriptive study. *Journal of Homosexuality*, 4(2): 123-141.

Fifield, L., Latham, D., & Phillips, C. (1977), *Alcoholism in the gay community: the price of alienation, isolation, and oppression*. Available from the Los Angeles Gay Community Center, Los Angeles, California.

Guze, S. (1976), *Criminality and psychiatric disorders*. New York: Oxford University Press, p. 34-35.

Kinsey, A., Pomeroy, W., & Martin, C. (1953), *Sexual behavior in the human female*. Philadelphia: Saunders.

Lewis, C., Saghir, M., Robins, E. (1982), Drinking patterns in homosexual and heterosexual women. *Journal of Clinical Psychiatry*, 43(7): 277-279.

Lohrenz, L., Connelly, J., Coyne, L., & Spare, K. (1978), Alcohol problems in several midwestern homosexual communities. *Journal of Studies on Alcohol*, 39(11): 1959-1963.

McKirnan, D., & Peterson, P. (1989), Alcohol and drug use among homosexual men and women: epidemiology and population characteristics. *Addictive Behaviors*, 14: 545-553.

Mischke, H., & Venneri, R. (1987), Reliability and validity of the MAST, Mortimer-Filkens questionnaire and CAGE in DWI assessment. *Journal of Studies on Alcohol*, 5: 492-501.

Moore, R. (1971), The prevalence of alcoholism in a community general hospital. *American Journal of Psychiatry*, 128: 638-639.

Moore, R. (1972), The diagnosis of alcoholism in a psychiatric hospital: a trial of the Michigan Alcoholism Screening Test. *American Journal of Psychiatry*, 128(12): 1565-1569.

Mosbacher, D. (1988), Lesbian alcohol and substance abuse. *Psychiatric Annals*, 18(1): 47-50.

Nardi, P. (1982), Alcoholism and homosexuality: a theoretical perspective. In *Alcoholism & Homosexuality*. Edited by Ziebold, T. & Mongeon, J. New York: The Haworth Press, Inc.

Nicoloff, L., & Stiglitz, E. (1987), Lesbian alcoholism: etiology, treatment, and recovery. In *Lesbian Psychologies*. Edited by The Boston Lesbian Psychologies Collective. Urbana and Chicago: University of Illinois Press.

Saghir, M., Robins, E., Walbran, B., & Gentry, K. (1970), Homosexuality. IV. psychiatric disorders and disability in the female homosexual. *American Journal of Psychiatry*, 127(2): 65-72.

Selzer, M. (1971), The Michigan Alcoholism Screening Test: the quest for a new diagnostic instrument. *American Journal of Psychiatry*, 127(12): 1653-1658.

Skinner, H., & Sheu, W. (1982), Reliability of alcohol use indices, the lifetime drinking history and the MAST. *Journal of Studies on Alcohol*, 43(11): 1157-1169.

Stevens (1986), *Applied multivariate statistics for the social sciences*. Lawrence Erlbaum Associates: New Jersey, 113-228.

Zung, B., & Charalampous, K. (1975), Item analysis of the Michigan Alcoholism Screening Test. *Journal of Studies on Alcohol*, 36(1): 127-132.

Gay Men, Lesbians
and Substances of Abuse
and the "Club and Circuit Party Scene":
What Clinicians Should Know

David McDowell, MD

SUMMARY. Many researchers believe that substance use rates are higher among gay men and lesbians than in the general population. In particular, recreational drugs, used as part of weekend and night "life" are particularly popular. In recent years these so called "club drugs" have become a regular part of many gay men and women's social life. MDMA, better known as "Ecstasy," is a synthetic amphetamine derivative, with some unique physiological properties. MDMA can induce depression and panic attacks in those who use it. A serious concern is the potential that MDMA may cause long lasting, even permanent neuropsychiatric damage, in particular to serotonin neurons. Ketamine, "Special K," is a dissasociative anesthetic which induces feelings of unreality, and may even cause catatonia (a "K hole"). GHB is a naturally occurring biological substance which has effects similar to alcohol. Modest doses can cause sleep, and coma. There have been a growing number of reports of fatal overdoses associated with GHB. The clinician working with gay and lesbian people is urged to become aware of these particular substances, as well as other recreational drugs, as well as their dangers, in order to more effectively work with his or her clients. *[Article copies available for a fee from The Haworth*

Dr. David McDowell is Assistant Professor of Clinical Psychiatry and Director, The Substance Treatment and Research Service (STARS), Columbia University/The New York State Psychiatric Institute, 600 West 168th Street, Second Floor, New York, NY 10032 (E-mail: dmm6@columbia.edu).

This article has been adapted, in part, from a chapter from the American Psychiatric Association Textbook on Substance Abuse Treatment: Marc Galanter and Herbert Kleber, Editors, APA Press, Washington DC.

[Haworth co-indexing entry note]: "Gay Men, Lesbians and Substances of Abuse and the 'Club and Circuit Party Scene': What Clinicians Should Know." McDowell, David. Co-published simultaneously in *Journal of Gay & Lesbian Psychotherapy* (The Haworth Medical Press, an imprint of The Haworth Press, Inc.) Vol. 3, No. 3/4, 2000, pp. 37-57; and: *Addictions in the Gay and Lesbian Community* (ed: Jeffrey R. Guss, and Jack Drescher) The Haworth Medical Press, an imprint of The Haworth Press, Inc., 2000, pp. 37-57. Single or multiple copies of this article are available from The Haworth Document Delivery Service [1-800-342-9678, 9:00 a.m. - 5:00 p.m. (EST). E-mail address: getinfo@haworthpressinc.com].

© 2000 by The Haworth Press, Inc. All rights reserved.

Document Delivery Service: 1-800-342-9678. E-mail address: <getinfo@haworth pressinc.com> Website: <http://www.HaworthPress.com>]

KEYWORDS. Club drugs, MDMA, Ecstasy, Ketamine, K hole, GHB, raves

Much has been written about substance abuse within the gay community. This is an extremely broad topic, and as varied as the individuals who use these drugs. Although there is scant hard evidence, most people who study these issues agree that rates of substance use are higher in gay and lesbian individuals than in the population in general (McDowell, 1999; Lee and McDowell, 1999). There are, however, some illicit substances that are especially popular among gay men and lesbians. A working knowledge of these substances, their history, chemistry, physiological effects, and the treatment options available is important for a clinician that works with this population.

Methylenedioxymethamphetamine (MDMA), Ketamine, and Gamma Hydroxybutyrate (GHB) are unique compounds, differing in terms of their pharmacological properties and their phenomenological effects. They are particularly popular within the gay community, and are, for some, an integral part of social life. They are not of course, the sole provinces of gay men and women, and individuals from quite varied backgrounds, and in many different ways use these drugs. They are particularly popular among young people who are part of the "rave" culture. With gays and lesbians, they are most often associated with nightclubs and circuit parties. Hence, these three drugs, which will be discussed extensively, and several others, which will be described more briefly, are widely known as "club drugs."

In recent years, the popularity of the "club drugs" has been inextricably linked with the rise of the "rave" phenomenon. Anecdotal reports suggest that raves were "created" in Ibiza, an island off the coast of Spain, known as a destination for Europeans and Americans interested in beaches and nightlife. Raves first became popular in England during the late 1980s and have since spread to the United States and the rest of the world. In the early 1990s, raves were considered "the next big thing," a rising trend. Although their popularity has not grown dramatically, it has remained relatively constant.

At raves, groups of young people (typically in their teens) dance to rapid electronically synthesized music with no lyrics (techno). These events traditionally take place in unregulated and unlicensed locations such as stadiums, abandoned warehouses, and other surreptitious arenas. There are significant numbers of individuals at these events who identify themselves as gay, lesbian or bisexual (McDowell and Kleber, 1994). Since the early nineties, the venues have become increasingly "mainstream." These drugs, along with marijuana and LSD, are extremely popular at these events. At some of these events, as many as 70% of rave participants are using Ecstasy, Ketamine, or GHB, along with other drugs like marijuana and LSD (McDowell and Kleber, 1994).

Circuit parties are large-scale social events, which have become increasingly popular among gay men over the last decade. At these events, several thousand people, mostly (but not exclusively) gay men, congregate in a dance club setting. Several of these events have been associated with fundraising events, in particular organizations which fund services and research concerned with HIV related disease.

These were, initially, small events that took place in private rather than commercial settings. Recently, they have become much larger, and spawned a worldwide industry, including a magazine called *Circuit Noize*, which is dedicated to issues related to circuit parties. These parties are held in various cities throughout the United States and in several countries including Australia, Canada, and Greece. These events typically take place over several days and involve numerous related events. Alcohol is often readily available at these events. There have been numerous anecdotal and media reports citing rampant and illicit drug use among attendees at circuit parties. One concern about the drug use at these parties is the possible toxicity of the drugs themselves. In the early morning hours before a New York area circuit party, one man died from a fatal overdose, and many speculate that his drug use was related to the atmosphere of permissiveness towards drugs associated with the circuit party (Bruni, 1998). Another concern is the possible increase in unsafe sex practices associated with intoxication.

MDMA

Introduction

Many groups, including HIV-organizations and gay and lesbian community groups, have used circuit parties as fund-raising events, raising hundreds of thousands of dollars in a single night. There is increasing controversy over the role of circuit parties as fund raisers. A popular circuit party held on Fire Island in the summer of 1998 raised $450,000 for AIDS research, but resulted in the death of at least one participant. MDMA has unique subjective and biochemical properties (Shulgin, 1986, Hermle, 1993). Recreational use of MDMA has been illegal since it was made a Schedule I drug on July 1, 1985. Prior to that time, because it was not mentioned in the controlled substances act of 1970, its use was unregulated and therefore legal. In spite of its illegal status, its use has skyrocketed in the past several years (Cohen, 1997). This rise in usage has been particularly marked among adolescents, and MDMA has been powerfully linked to raves. It is also sometimes known as a "gay drug" because of its popularity at gay bars and nightclubs.

MDMA damages brain serotonin neurons in laboratory animals (McCann,

1993). Although it is not definitively known if MDMA is neurotoxic to humans, the weight of current scientific evidence indicate that this is probably the case (Gold, 1997). A recent article by McCann (1998) compared subjects with extensive use of MDMA to matched controls. The MDMA users had significantly less serotonin activity as measured using Positron Emission Tomography (PET). The indirect implication is that the use of MDMA is indeed neurotoxic. This is particularly germane for individuals with affective illness. Lower serotonin levels correspond with depression and impulsivity. Individuals who are prone to or have a history of depression and anxiety are warned to use MDMA with particular caution.

MDMA's appeal rests primarily on its psychological effect, a dramatic and consistent induction in the user, a profound feeling of attachment and connection. This feeling of connection is not necessarily to another individual, and people who use the drug alone may feel "connected to" the larger world. The compound is perhaps a misnomer; the LA dealer who coined the term Ecstasy, wanted to call the drug "Empathy," but asked, "who would know what that means?" (Eisner, 1986).

History

MDMA is not a new drug. It was first patented in 1914 by Merck in Darmstadt, Germany (Shulgin, 1990). MDMA was probably patented as so many compounds were at that time, to serve for subsequent research. Except for a minor chemical modification in a patent in 1919, there is no other known historical record of MDMA until the 1950s. At that time, the United States Army experimented with MDMA. The resulting informational material was declassified and became available to the general public in the early 1970s. These findings consisted primarily of a number of Lethal Dose determinations for a variety of laboratory animals. MDMA was apparently not used on humans at that time.

MDMA was first used by humans, probably in the late 1960s. It was lionized as a recreational drug by free thinkers and "New Age Seekers," people who liked its properties of inducing feelings of well being and connection (Watson, 1991). Given MDMA's capacity to induce feelings of warmth and openness, a number of practitioners and researchers interested in insight-oriented psychotherapy believed it would be an ideal agent to enhance the therapeutic process (Shulgin, 1990). Before use of the compound became illegal in 1985, it was used extensively for this purpose (Beck, 1990). There are a number of uncontrolled case series by practitioners who used the drug for this purpose.

In the early 1980s, MDMA became increasingly popular. The drug's capacity to induce feelings of connection, as well as a psychomotor agitation that can be pleasurably relieved by dancing, made it the ideal "party drug." In spite of widespread usage during the early 1980s, the drug did not attract much attention from the media, or from law enforcement officials. This is not particularly surprising in that individuals on the drug tend to be complacent and do not exhibit the kind of behavior likely to attract the attention of the police.

Events in Texas, especially in the Dallas/Fort Worth area changed this lack of notoriety. Until 1985, the drug was not scheduled or regulated and its use was legal. A distribution network in Texas began an aggressive marketing campaign and, for a time, the drug was available over the counter at bars, at convenience stores, and even through a toll-free number. This widespread distribution attracted the attention of then Texas Senator Lloyd Bentsen (the future vice presidential candidate, and Secretary of the Treasury). He petitioned the FDA, and the compound was placed on Schedule I on an emergency basis as of July 1, 1985. Originally, three hearings were scheduled to determine MDMA's permanent scheduling status. FDA officials were reportedly surprised that a substantial number of people, including therapists and clergymen, came out in support of a less restrictive categorization. The compound's possible neurotoxicity, combined with concern about illicit drug use in general, resulted in MDMA's permanent placement on Schedule I, which refers to substances that have no therapeutic value, and which are considered to have high abuse potential. Its clinical use is therefore prohibited, and because of the intense regulation of Schedule I compounds, research with MDMA is technically possible, but almost impossible to execute. It remains on Schedule I today, and although there are some individuals who believe the drug should be more widely available for research, its status will not likely change in the foreseeable future (Cohen, 1997).

The chemical synthesis of MDMA is relatively simple, and it is often made in illicit laboratories, or even domestic locations such as garages. In addition, it is often cut with other substances so the purity and dosage varies substantially. It currently sells in urban areas for about $25 to $30 per 125 mg tablet, which produces the sought after effect in most intermittent users (Green et al., 1995).

Physiological Effects

Tablets of MDMA are usually ingested orally. Other methods of administration are much less popular, and virtually unheard of. The usual single dose is between 100-150 mg. The onset of effect begins about 20-40 minutes after ingestion and is experienced as a sudden, amphetamine-like "rush." Nausea, usually mild, but sometimes severe enough to cause vomiting, often accompanies this initial feeling. In addition sometimes the intense desire to defecate (known as a "disco dump") accompanies this initial phase.

The reason to take the drug, according to most users, is a profound feeling of relatedness to the rest of the world. This accompanies the plateau stage of drug effects which last between three and four hours. Most users experience this feeling as a powerful connection to those around them, and this may include the larger world. In general, people on the drug appear to be less aggressive, and less impulsive than their counterparts. Users also experience an altered perception of time and a decreased inclination to perform mental and physical tasks (Leister et al., 1992). Although the desire for sex can increase, the ability to achieve arousal and orgasm for men and women is greatly diminished (Buffem, 1986). It has thus been termed a sensual, not a sexual, drug. In addition, people on the drug have mild psychomotor restlessness as well as teeth grinding, jaw clenching, anorexia, sweating, hot flashes, tremor and "goose bumps" (Paroutka, 1988). The array of physical effects and behaviors produced by MDMA is remarkably similar across mammalian species (Green et al., 1995).

Common after-effects can be pronounced, typically lasting 24 hours. The most dramatic "hangover" effect is a sometimes-severe feeling of depression and listlessness. Users of MDMA can experience lethargy, anorexia, decreased motivation, sleepiness, depressed mood and fatigue, occasionally lasting for days. There are a few cases of more severe consequences of MDMA use. These include altered mental status, convulsions, hypo- or hyperthermia, severe changes in blood pressure, tachycardia, coagulopathies, acute renal failure, hepatotoxicity as well as death (Demirkiran et al., 1996).

There are numerous case reports of a single dose of MDMA precipitating severe psychiatric illness. MDMA probably does induce a range of depressive symptoms and anxiety in some individuals, and for that reason people with affective illness should be specifically cautioned about the dangers of using MDMA (McCann et al., 1994). Many of these reports represent single cases and there are often other potential explanations for these occurrences. Still, the growing number of such adverse events is cause for concern.

Mechanism of Action

MDMA is a "dirty drug," because it affects both serotonin and dopamine-containing neurons, as well as a host of other neurotransmitter systems (Rattray, 1991). MDMA's primary mechanism of action is as an indirect serotonergic agonist (Ames, 1993). MDMA is taken up by the serotonin cell through an active channel where it induces the release of stored serotonin. The drug also blocks re-uptake of serotonin, contributing to its length of action. (It also inhibits further synthesis, but this effect probably does not contribute to the intoxicating effects.) It may however, contribute to sustained feelings of depression reported by some users, and diminished magnitude of subjective effects if the next dose is taken within a few days of the first dose. The drug's various side effects including anorexia, psychomotor agitation, difficulty in achieving orgasm, and profound feelings of empathy, can all be explained as a result of the flooding of the serotonin system (Beck, 1994).

Unlike other substances of abuse, where escalating dosage and frequency are common, people who use MDMA on a regular basis tend not to use more and more of the substance as time goes on (Paroutka, 1990). Because the drug depletes serotonin stores and inhibits synthesis of new serotonin; subsequent doses produce a diminished "high" and a worsening of the drug's undesirable effects. People who use the drug quickly become aware of this consequence and adjust their usage patterns. Many users who are at first enamored with the drug, subsequently lose interest, usually citing the substantial side effects. It is rare to find someone who uses the drug frequently, over the course of years. There is an adage on college campuses about Ecstasy which captures this phenomenon: "Freshmen love it, sophomores like it, Juniors are ambivalent, and Seniors are afraid of it" (Eisner, 1993). Those who continue to use the drug over longer periods of time usually tend to use the drug only periodically. It is therefore reserved for "special occasions." Many gay men report "saving" their ecstasy use for special occasions, especially for the more major circuit parties.

The drug's effects can be characterized as short term (< 24 hours) and long term (> 24 hours) (McKenna and Peroutka, 1990). The short-term effects (the high) are presumably due to acute release of serotonin (5-HT) and are associated with a decrease in 5-HT and 5 hydoxyinodoleacetic acid (5-HIAA), a decrease in tryptamine hydoxylase (TPH) activity, and recovery of 5-HIAA levels usually within 24 hours. The long-term effects are manifested by persistent slow decrease in 5-HT and 5-HIAA after initial recovery, persistently depressed TPH activity, and a decrease in 5-HT terminal density (Demirkiran et al., 1996).

In the summer of 1992, there were as many as fifteen deaths, associated with the use of MDMA in England. These deaths all occurred at raves. These deaths appear to be similar to certain features of both the Serotonin (5-HT) Syndrome and the Neuroleptic Malignant Syndrome (Ames and Wirshing, 1993). The "Serotonin Syndrome" is a clinical phenomenon which occurs with an excess of the neurotransmitter serotonin and is characterized by confusion, restlessness, hyperthermia, diaphoresis, hyper-reflexia, diarrhea, and myoclonus (Sternback, 1991). The Neuroleptic Malignant Syndrome (NMS) is associated with the use of antipsychotics (dopamine blockers) and dehydration and consists of mental status changes, hyperthermia, rigidity, elevated CK, and autonomic dysfunction (Guerra et al., 1992). Both syndromes exist on a spectrum of severity, but in their most severe form they are life threatening.

Raves are often held in hot, crowded conditions. During the summer of 1992, some of the clubs turned off their water supplies in an effort to maximize profits by selling bottled water. The hot, crowded conditions, physical exertion, and subsequent dehydration combined with the drug effects certainly contributed to the deaths. After these incidents, the English government mandated an open water supply at all clubs; deaths of this kind appear to have since diminished, though they do still occur (Demirikiran et al., 1996). In recent years, one of the principal aims of the harm reduction efforts in England aimed at young people who take the drug is to remind them that if they are going to take the drug, they must keep well hydrated.

Although rare, there have been anecdotal reports of MDMA causing Post Hallucinogenic Perception Disorder (Creighton et al. 1991). This disorder is a prolonged re-experience of the perceptual distortion produced during the MDMA "high." Post Hallucinogenic Perceptual Disorder is more commonly associated with LSD ingestion, and can last for months, even years. Although symptoms tend to diminish over time, there are no effective treatments for this disorder. The literature on this disorder is scant, but most reports indicate that the symptoms eventually diminish without treatment. A calm "wait and see" attitude is therefore advised if this occurs.

MDMA and Neurotoxicity

In laboratory animals, the ingestion of MDMA causes a decrease in the serum and spinal fluid levels of 5-HIAA in a dose-dependent fashion (Shulgin, 1990) and damages brain serotonin neurons (McCann, 1993). The dose levels necessary to cause permanent damage to most of the rodent species is many times greater than that normally ingested by humans (Shulgin, 1990). In non-human primates, the neurotoxic dose approximates the recreational dose taken by humans (McCann, 1993). Like its close structural relative MDA, MDMA has been found to damage serotonin neurons in all animal species tested to date (McCann et al., 1996). The closer phylogenetically to humans a given mammal is, the less MDMA is required to induce this permanent damage.

Unequivocal data demonstrating that similar changes occur in the human brain do not exist, but the indirect clinical evidence is disconcerting (Green, 1995). MDMA users have significantly less serotonin metabolites in their spinal fluid than matched controls (McCann, 1998). Clear deficits and major neurotoxicity appear to be related to total cumulative dose in animals (Gold et al., 1997). In addition, MDMA produces a 30-35% drop in 5-HT metabolism in humans (McCann et al., 1994). It is possible that even one dose of MDMA may cause lasting damage to the serotonin system. Furthermore, such damage might only become apparent with time, or under conditions of stress. Users with no initial complications may manifest problems over time (McCann et al., 1996). There have been reports of individuals with lasting neuropsychiatric disturbances after MDMA use (Creighton, 1991, McCann, 1991, Shifano, 1991).

The clinical impact of serotonergic damage is not clear since some animal data suggest that even significant destruction of serotonin neurons leads to little functional impairment (Robinson et al., 1993). Whether this holds true for humans is unclear, however. Until the full impact of widespread MDMA use is known, the risks must be taken seriously. The drug's potential neurotoxicity is the most significant concern about its use. The drug may be particularly attractive to gay individuals who complain of disenfranchisement, but the costs may be great.

Treatment

MDMA intoxication, adverse reactions, and permanent sequalae may require treatment. As discussed previously, dehydration, coupled with the direct effects of MDMA may be life threatening. The clinical characteristics of these cases resemble a combination of the Serotonin Syndrome and the Neuroleptic Malignant Syndrome (NMS). It should therefore be treated in the emergency room as if the patient has both these conditions. This is an uncommon, but potentially fatal occurrence. The treatment recommendations that follow are adopted from the standard treatment given patients with NMS (Kaplan and Saddock, 1995, Bernstein, 1996).

Clinicians should be alert to the possibility of these syndromes in any patient who presents with confusion or impaired sensorium, hyperthermia, muscle rigidity, and fever. If it can be established that a patient has been to a rave, or some gay club or circuit party, this should raise the suspicion that MDMA was ingested. This is a diagnosis of exclusion, other disorders must first be ruled out. These include infections such as meningitis, trauma, and other drug intoxications. Management should include consultation with a trained neurologist and transfer to the Intensive Care Unit as quickly as possible. Supportive measures such as effective hydration using intravenous fluids and lowering the temperature of the patient with cooling blankets or an ice bath are often necessary. Standard gastric lavage should be utilized. When other diagnoses have been excluded, the clinician should consider treating the patient with the medications that are commonly used to treat both traditional NMS and the Serotonin Syndrome.

MDMA intoxication is associated with a number of psychiatric symptoms, particularly anxiety, panic, and depression. These are usually short-term sequelae and subside in a matter of days. Support and reassurance are often all that is needed to help the individual through this difficult time. If the symptoms are severe, brief pharmacotherapy, probably with a benzodiazepine, is recommended.

Although physiological dependence on MDMA does not occur, there are certainly individuals who use the drug compulsively and can be said to be dependent upon it. For them, the standard approaches utilized in substance abuse are recommended. These patients can be difficult to treat for many reasons. They are usually gay men who are heavily involved in the club culture (McDowell and Spitz, 1999). Getting such an individual to abandon their way of socializing may be a daunting task. Another complicating factor is that MDMA, as compared to other drugs, is often viewed as benign (Beck, 1994). As a result, there is little urgency among either the gay culture or general public to eradicate MDMA as compared to other drugs with more negative reputations.

KETAMINE

Introduction

Ketamine was first manufactured in 1965, and is still legally produced, primarily for use by veterinarians and pediatric surgeons as a non-analgesic anesthetic. It is variously known as Special K, Super K, Vitamin K or just plain K. Supplies from these sources are frequently diverted to recreational users. The recreational use of Ketamine in humans probably began soon after Ketamine was available. John Lilly (1978) first described it in detail. Since that time its popularity has continued to rise (Dotson et al., 1995; Cooper, 1996).

Ketamine is an anesthetic agent that induces dissociation. As its name implies, the drug causes a dose-dependent dissociative episode with feelings of fragmentation, detachment, a feeling of disconnection. It induces a lack of responsive awareness not only to pain but to the general environment as well, without a corresponding depression of autonomic reflexes in various parts of the Central Nervous System.

History

Ketamine was first manufactured in 1965 at the University of Michigan. It was first available in the brand name Ketalar, by the pharmaceutical firm Parke-Davis. Since that time it has been commercially available under a variety of brand names. It is most commonly available in 10-ml. liquid containing vials, containing 100 mg/ml (Fort Dodge, 1997). It is quite similar in mechanism and action to PCP, but offers a number of distinct advantages.

PCP also had a number of severe limitations as an anesthetic, most significantly that it causes frequent psychotic and violent reactions (NIDA, 1979). At least half of the patients subjected to PCP anesthesia developed several perioperative reactions, including agitation and hallucinations. While it was being studied and used as an anesthetic, some of these people developed severe psychotic reactions which persisted for as long as 240 hours (Crider, 1986; Meyer, 1959). Clinically, these problems are much less severe with the use of Ketamine. Ketamine produces minimal cardiac and respiratory effects and its anesthetic and behavioral effects remit soon after administration (Pandit et al., 1980; Moretti et al., 1984). The medication has a limited place in the pharmacopoeia of anesthesia, principally with children and animals.

Like so many other drugs, Ketamine has been popular with a number of different types of users; these can be conveniently divided into two different subsets. The first type of user takes ketamine in a solitary fashion and seeks a paranormal experience or uses it to enhance a spiritual journey. The second type uses the drug at social gatherings. Ketamine is especially popular at "circuit parties." Epidemiological evidence about the use of Ketamine is difficult to obtain. Reports in the media, anecdotal evidence, and observations by the author while treating patients indicate that Ketamine is quite popular in urban clubs and at raves. At a recent circuit party held in the New York area, over 50% of the participants surveyed indicated that they had used Ketamine that day (Lee and McDowell, 1999).

Ketamine is sold commercially as a liquid. The liquid form is easily converted to a powder. At clubs and through dealers, Ketamine is most commonly sold in this form. Ketamine can be administered in a variety of ways. In its most potent form, it is mixed with water and injected. Because of aversions to IV use, this is probably not the most popular form. At clubs, most people snort lines of the powder. Ketamine may also be dabbed on the tongue or mixed with a liquid and taken orally.

Physiological Effects

Ketamine has been studied extensively in humans, both as an anesthetic and as a drug of abuse. Not surprisingly, recreational users of Ketamine report feeling anesthetized and sedated. The intensity of this feeling is a dose-dependent phenomenon (Krystal et al., 1994). For example, relatively low Ketamine can induce tangential thinking and ideas of reference. At higher doses, it distorts perception of the body, the environment, and time. Ketamine influences all modes of sensory function (Oye et al., 1992). At typical doses, Ketamine distorts sensory stimuli, producing illusions (Garfield et al., 1972). In higher than typical doses, hallucinations and paranoid delusions can occur (Malhotra et al., 1996). Attention and learning are substantially affected by the use of Ketamine. This has been amply demonstrated in research volunteers. Individuals on Ketamine take longer to learn initial tasks and do not apply strategy. A variety of memory functions is affected by Ketamine: retrieval, long-term recall, and the consolidation of memory are all altered (Krystal et al., 1994).

Ketamine has a relatively high therapeutic index. The lethal dose is nearly thirty times the anesthetic dose. According to users, the minimal risk of overdosing is one of the attractive properties of the drug. The recreational dose is approximately 0.4 mg per kg; the anesthetic dose is almost double that. Tolerance to Ketamine develops rapidly.

Individuals injecting the drug recreationally begin to feel the effects in about five minutes. Intra-nasal users experience the effects of the drug in about ten minutes. While there are initial tingling sensations and mild effects that occur almost immediately, the principle dissociative effect occurs about ten minutes later. In the first half-hour after ingestion, the peak effects of the drug occur and then gradually subside. The bulk of the "trip" lasts about an hour (Delgarno & Shewan, 1996). This is known as the emergence state, and it is here that the perception of time is significantly altered. Users describe a sense of "eternity" and a heightened capacity to discern causal connections in all things. The effects gradually diminish over another hour. Larger doses last longer and have a more intense effect (Malhotra, 1996). Flashbacks have been reported, and their incidence may be higher than in hallucinogens (Seigel and Jarvik, 1975).

An observer of someone who has recently used Ketamine may notice catatonia, a flat face, an open mouth, fixed staring with dilated pupils, "sightless staring," rigid posturing, and waxy flexibility. At higher doses, the user enters a catatonic state colloquially known as a "K hole."

Social withdrawal, autistic behavior, an inability to think clearly, impoverished and idiosyncratic thought patterns, and bizarre responses characterize the catatonic state induced by Ketamine use. Motor impairment is a marked feature of this state, and people in a "K-hole" are found on the edge of the dance floor, staring blankly into space, appearing non-distressed, but seemingly incapable of communication (GMHC, 1997).

Mechanism of Action

Molecular mechanisms underlying Ketamine effects have recently been identified. Ketamine interferes with the actions of the excitatory amino acid neurotransmitters especially glutamate and aspartate, the most prevalent excitatory neurotransmitters in the brain. These regulate numerous functions of the central nervous system and are particularly important in cortical-cortical and cortical-subcortical interactions (Cotman, 1987). The excitatory amino acid receptor subtype which Ketamine binds to with the most affinity is the N-methyl-D-Aspartate (NMDA) receptor complex, which regulates calcium flow through its ion channel. Ketamine binds to the NMDA receptor complex on the same site as Phencyclidine, located inside the calcium channel. Therefore the direct action of Ketamine is the blockade of calcium movement through this channel (Hampton, 1982).

Noncompetitive antagonism of NMDA receptors by the "channel blockers" is known to induce changes of perception, memory, and cognition throughout the brain. In addition, the channel blockers have been shown to affect dopaminergic transmission, inhibiting cocaine-induced increases in extra-cellular dopamine in the nucleus accumbens (Pap & Bradberry, 1995).

NMDA blockade causes an increase in dopamine release in the mid-brain and pre-frontal cortex (Bubser, 1992). NMDA blockade also causes activation of 5-HT systems specifically targeting the 5-HT1A receptor (Loscher and Ha-nock, 1993). Agents such as Ketamine clearly work globally, directly or indirectly affecting numerous neurotransmitter systems. Nonetheless, the principal effects of Ketamine appear to result from its actions as an NMDA antagonist.

Treatment

Because of its high therapeutic index, only cases of severe overdose present substantial risk of significant morbidity and mortality. These rare cases should be treated in the Intensive Care Unit. Perhaps the most dangerous effects of Ketamine are behavioral. Individuals may become withdrawn, paranoid, and very uncoordinated. In such a case, the treating physician must treat the patient symptomatically. Usually calm reassurance and a low stimulation environment is most helpful. Clinical experience indicates that less stimulation is better. The person should be placed in a part of the clinic or emergency room with the least amount of light and stimulation. Neuroleptics should be used in only the rarest of cases, because their side effect profile may cause discomfort and therefore provoke the patient. If necessary, the individual may be given benzodiazepines for control of the associated anxiety.

Ketamine is an addictive drug. It is reinforcing in the classical sense. There are numerous reports of individuals who become dependent upon the drug and use it on a daily basis (Galloway, 1997). Such individuals ought to be treated in the traditional manner. The clinician should evaluate the patient for any underlying psychiatric condition, and if such a condition is not found, then individual treatment should focus on the drug use issues.

GHB

Introduction

GHB, or gamma-hydroxybutyrate, is sold as "liquid Ecstasy" and in Britain, as GBH, or "grievous bodily harm." (They apparently are not upset about the change in word order.) It is found naturally in many mammalian cells, and some consider it a neurotransmitter (Galloway, 1997). In the mammalian brain, the highest amounts are found in the hypothalamus and basal ganglia (Gallimberti, 1989). GHB is closely linked to Gamma Amino Butyric Acid, an inhibitory neurotransmitter. GHB, however, does not act directly on GABA receptor sites (Chin and Kreutzer, 1992).

In some European countries, GHB is available by prescription. Most of the GHB sold in this country is manufactured by nonprofessional "kitchen" chemists, in an illicit fashion. In fact, it is reportedly easy to manufacture, and there are a number of Internet sites that explain the process. The unregulated nature of these operations arouses concern about the quality and safety of the GHB available to recreational users.

In the seventies, GHB did not receive much attention when it was used as a sleep aid. It is effective for this, and has been used in the treatment of narcolepsy (Scrima, 1992, Lammers, 1993). In addition, body builders sometimes still use it, hoping it will promote muscle growth, because it increases episodic secretion of growth hormone. There is scant evidence for efficacy in this regard, but it does increase the production of growth hormone. In 1990, after reports indicated that GHB may have contributed to the hospitalization of several California youths, its sale and manufacture were banned by the FDA. It has not been scheduled by the DEA as a drug, however, so possession of it is legal. The law prohibits GHB being manufactured for sale to laboratories for research purposes, sale to the public, or the manufacture of it with this intent. The chief danger involved with GHB is that it has an extremely small therapeutic index, and as little as double the euphorigenic dose may cause serious CNS depression. In recent years, it has been associated with several incidents of respiratory depression and coma. In the late 1990s, there have been several deaths linked to GHB. Furthermore it is ingested as a liquid, and can be easily put into someone's drink surreptitiously.

History

Dr. H. Laborit, a French scientist who was investigating the effects of GABA on the mammalian brain, first synthesized GHB over thirty years ago. Laborit was attempting to manufacture a GABA-like agent which would cross the blood-brain barrier (Vickers, 1969). In this regard he succeeded. It was studied as a sleep aid in the 1970s but there were much more efficacious (and safe) alternatives. During the 1980s, GHB was widely available over-the-counter in health food stores. It came to the attention of regulatory authorities in the late 1980s as a potential drug of abuse, and after reports of several poisonings associated with GHB, the FDA banned it in 1990 (Chin and Kreutzer, 1992). In the past decade, it has become more widely known as a drug of abuse associated with nightclubs and raves. It is popular at Circuit Parties and other nightclubs frequented by gays and lesbians.

Psychological Effects

GHB is ingested orally, rapidly absorbed, and reaches peak plasma concentrations in 20 to 60 minutes (Vickers, 1969). The typical recreational dose is between 0.75 and 1.5 gm, with higher doses resulting in increased effects. The "high" lasts for no more than 90 minutes and reportedly, has few lasting effects. Repeated use of the drug can prolong its effects. Tolerance develops, and it can be quite robust.

Users of the drug report that GHB induces a pleasant state of relaxation and tranquillity. Frequently reported effects are placidity, mild euphoria, and a tendency to verbalize. One patient, who reported using it, described feeling "cat like." GHB, like MDMA, has also been described as a sensual drug. Its effects have been likened to alcohol, another GABA-like drug (McCabe et al., 1971).

There is some cross-reactivity with alcohol, and in combination this can be dangerous, and even lethal. Users report a feeling of mild numbing, and pleasant disinhibition. This disinhibition is the likely desired effect, and responsible for the drug's reputation of being effective for sex. The dose response curve for GHB is exceedingly steep. The recommended or intoxicating dose can result in severe adverse effects. The LD-50 is estimated at perhaps only 5 times the intoxicating dose (Vickers, 1971). Furthermore, the drug has synergistic effects with alcohol and probably other drugs as well. Therefore, small increases in the amount ingested may lead to significant intensification of the effects as well as the onset of CNS depression. Overdose is a real and significant danger. Those drinking alcohol are at greater risk. The reasons for this are two fold: alcohol is synergistic with GHB, and those drinking exhibit impaired judgement and may be more prone to overdose.

Commonly reported side effects associated with GHB ingestion are drowsiness, dizziness, nausea, and vomiting. Less common side effects include weakness, loss of peripheral vision, confusion, agitation, hallucinations, and bradycardia. The drug is a sedative and can produce loss of coordination, and difficulty ambulating. As the dose ingested increases, patients may experience loss of bladder control, temporary amnesia, and sleepwalking. Clonus, as well as cardiopulmonary depression can occur. Coma and persistent vegetative states have been reported. Seizures have been reported, but it is unclear if this is a true effect of GHB, or whether this is the result of a mislabeling of the effect of clonus (Chin and Kreutzer, 1992; Gallimberti, 1989; Takahara, 1977; Vickers, 1969).

Mechanism of Action

It is likely that GHB is a neurotransmitter, although the function in situ is far from clear (Galloway, 1997). Specific high-affinity binding sites for GHB have been found in the rat brain (Hechler, 1992). GHB temporarily suppresses the release of dopamine in the mammalian brain. This is followed by a marked increase in dopamine release, especially in the nigro-striatal pathway, and is accompanied by the increased release of endogenous opioids (Hechler, 1990). This dopamine release is likely responsible for at least some of the euphorigenic properties.

GHB has a number of endocrine effects. GHB stimulates pituitary growth hormone (GH) release. One study (Takahara, 1977) reported nine-fold and sixteen-fold increases in growth hormone 30 and 60 minutes respectively after intravenous administration of 2.5 grams of GHB in six healthy adult men. The mechanism by which GHB stimulates GH release is not known. GHB induces serum Prolactin levels to rise, in a similar time-dependent fashion. GHB has several different actions in the CNS, and there are some reports that indicate it antagonizes marijuana's effects (Galloway, 1997). The consequences of these physiological changes are unclear. It is not at all known what the effects are on individuals who use the drug over a lengthy period of time.

Treatment

Clinicians should remember to ask about GHB in their gay patients who attend clubs, and who may be using it, and be unaware of the dangers of overdose. The fact that GHB is not detectable by routine drug screening makes this history that much more important. It can be detected, but only with the use of a specialized screen. In cases of acute GHB intoxication, physicians should provide physiological support and maintain a high index of suspicion for intoxication with other drugs. That is, if the patient is using GHB, he or she is likely to be on another drug. Often the most dangerous effects of GHB use have occurred with the use of other drugs. For example, concurrent use of sedatives or alcohol may increase the risk of vomiting, aspiration, or cardiopulmonary depression. These can be life threatening. The use of GHB and methamphetamine cocaine may increase the risk of seizure. When having received proper medical attention, most cases of GHB overdose have resulted in full recovery.

There are reports of individuals who have developed physiological dependence to GHB. The symptoms of withdrawal include anxiety, tremor, insomnia and "feelings of doom" which may persist for several weeks after stopping the drug (Galloway, 1997). There are anecdotal reports of even more severe dependence and withdrawal, sometimes lasting for days or weeks, and resembling severe alcohol withdrawal (Kato, personal communication). There are no studies that have examined the treatment of GHB withdrawal. This complex of symptomatology however, suggests that benzodiazepines may be useful in treating GHB withdrawal. Due to a lack of data, however, clinicians must exercise their most prudent judgment regarding what will be most helpful in a given situation. Health care professionals should be alert for abuse and overdose of this potentially dangerous drug.

CONCLUSION

The three drugs discussed above are by no means the only ones found at clubs, raves, or circuit parties. They are also not the only ones favored by gay men and lesbians. They are also not the sole provinces of gay and lesbian aficionados. They are, however, quite prominently used by at least a subset of gay men and lesbians. Club goers and those "on the circuit" also use more "traditional" drugs such as LSD, and other hallucinogens. Marijuana is perennially popular, and alcohol use is also high (Lee and McDowell, 1999). Recently, some drug users have begun to experiment with Flunitrazepam, a short acting benzodiazepine better known by its street name "Rohypnol," "Roofies," or "Ro." Because of the ability of this drug to interfere with short-term memory, it has become known in the media as "the date rape drug." (A name also applied to GHB.) Slipped into the drink of someone unsuspecting, it may indeed make the person feel very disinhibited and unable to remember much of what happened after ingestion. It is similar in action to short term benzodiazepines used in anesthesia. These drugs are used at clubs, often in combination, and often by very young people. This is cause for concern for several reasons. The younger a person begins using drugs, and the more often, the more likely he or she is to develop serious problems with these or other substances. This is especially true for gay youth who may be under more stress than their counterparts, and may be more at risk of substance abuse, and the dangers that accompany indiscriminate ingestion in an attempt to "fit in." Drugs and alcohol are not only a problem among gay men and women; much of society has problems with these substances. They are however quite visible in the gay and lesbian community. In the future we are likely to see more and more use of such drugs, and the problems that come with their use. The clinician working with this population should be aware of these substances and has an obligation to educate people about them.

REFERENCES

Ames D., Wirshing W. (1993), Ecstasy, the Serotonin Syndrome, and Neuroleptic Malignant Syndrome–a possible link? *JAMA*, 269 (7): 869-870.

Beck, J. & Rosenbaum, M. (1994), *Pursuit of Ecstasy: The MDMA experience.* SUNY Series in New Social Studies on Alcohol and Drugs. New York, NY: State University of New York Press.

Beck J. (1990), *The Public Health Implications of MDMA Use in Ecstasy: the Clinical, Pharmacological and Neurotoxicological Effects of the drug MDMA.* Edited by Peroutka, S.: Klewer Academic Publishing.

Bernstein C., Ladds B., Maloney A., & Weiner, E. (1997), *On Call Psychiatry.* Philadelphia: W.B. Saunders Company.

Bubser M., Keseberg U., Notz P.K., & Schmidt W.J. (1992), Differential behavioral and neurochemical effects of competitive and noncompetitive NMDA receptor antagonists in rats. *European Journal Pharmacology*, 229: 75-82.

Buffum J., & Moser C. (1986), MDMA and human sexual function. *J Psychoactive Drugs,* 18(4): 355-359.

Chin M.Y., Kreutzer R.A., & Dyer J.E. (1992), Acute poisoning from gamma-hydroxybutyrate in California. *West J Med*, 156(4): 380-384.

Corsessen G. & Domino E.F. (1966), Dissociative anesthesia: further pharmacologic studies and first clinical experience with the phencyclidine derivative CI-581. *Anesth Analg*, 45: 29-40.

Collins V.J., Gorrspe C.A., & Rovenstine, E.A. (1960), Intravenous nonbariburate nonnarcotic analgesics: preliminary studies. I Cychohexlamines. *Anesth Analg*, 39: 303-306.

Cohen, R. (1998), *The Love Drug: Marching to the Beat of Ecstasy.* Binghamton, NY: The Haworth Press, Inc.

Cooper, M. (Jan 28, 1996), "Special K: rough catnip for clubgoers." *New York Times*, p. 6.

Cotman C.W. & Monaghan D.T. (1987), Chapter 4. *Chemistry and anatomy of excitatory amino acid systems in Psychopharmacology: The Third Generation of Progress.* Edited by Meltzer HY, New York, NY: Raven Publishers, pp. 112-134.

Creighton F., Black D., & Hyde C. (1991), Ecstasy psychosis and flashbacks. *Br J Psychiatry*, 159: 713-715.

Crider R. (1986), Phencyclidine: changing abuse patterns. *NIDA Research Monograph*, 64: 163-173.

Demirkiran M., Jankovic J., & Dean J. (1996), Ecstasy Intoxication: An overlap between Serotonin Syndrome and Neuroleptic Malignant Syndrome. *Clin Neuropharmacology* 19(2): 157-164.

Delgarno P.J. & Shewan D. (1996), Illicit use of ketamine in Scotland. *J. Psychoactive Drugs*, 28: 191-199.

Dotson, J., Ackerman D., & West L. (1995), Ketamine Abuse. *Journal of Drug Issues*, 25(4): 751-757.

Eisner B. (1986), *Ecstasy: the MDMA Story.* Little Brown Publishers.

Fort Dodge Laboratories (1997), Ketaset® package insert. Fort Dodge Iowa, Ketamine HCL INJ USP.

Galloway G.P., Frederick S.L., Staggers F.E., Gonzales M., Stalcup A.S., & Smith D.E. (1997), Gamma-Hydroxybuturate: an emerging drug of abuse that causes physical dependence. *Addiction*, 92(1): 89-96.

Gallimberti L., Gentile N., Cibin M., Fadda F., Canton G., Ferri M., Ferrara S.D., & Gessa G.L. (1989), Gamma-hydroxybutyric acid for treatment of alcohol withdrawal syndrome. *Lancet*, 30: 787-789.

Garfield J.M., Garfield F.B., Stone J.G., Hopkins K., & Johns L.A. (1994), A comparison of psychologic responses to ketamine and thiopental-nitrous oxide-halothane anesthesia. *Anesthesiolgy*, 36: 329-338.

GMHC (McDowell, D., consultant) (1997), "Drugs in Partyland." educational brochure published by GMHC press.

Green A., Cross A., & Goodwin G. (1995), Review of pharmacology and clinical pharmacology of 3,4-methylenedioxymehtamphetamine (MDMA or "Ecstasy"). *Psychopharmacology*, 119: 247-260.

Guerra R., Chang S., & Romero J. (1992), A comparison of diagnostic criteria for neuroleptic malignant syndrome. *J Clin Psychiatry*, 53: 56-62.

Hampton R.Y., Medzihradsky F., Woods J.H., & Dahlstrom P.J. (1982), Stereospecific binding of 3H phencyclidine in Brain Membranes. *Life Science*, 30: 2147-2154.

Hechler V., Goebaille S., & Maitre M. (1992), Selective distribution pattern of gamma-hydroxybutyrate receptors in the rat forebrain and mid-brain as revealed by quantitative autoradiograph. *Brain Research*, 572: 345-348.

Hermle L., Spitzer M., Borchardt K., & Gouzoulis E. (1993), Psychological effects of MDE in normal subjects. *Neuropsychopharmacology*, 8(2): 171-76.

Henry J., Jeffrey K., & Dawling S. (1992), Toxicity and deaths from 3,4-methylenedioxymethamphetamine ("ecstasy"). *Lancet*, 340: 384-387.

Kaplan & Sadock, editors (1995), *The Comprehensive Textbook of Psychiatry: Sixth Edition*. Williams and Wilkins. Baltimore Md.

Krystal J.H., Karper L.P., Seityl J.P., Freeman G.K., Delaney R., Bremmer J.D., Heninger G.R., Bowers M.B., & Charney D.S. (1994), Subanesthetic effects of the noncompetitive NMDA antagonist ketamine in humans. *Arch Gen Psychiatry*, 51: 199-214.

Leister M., Grob C., Bravo G., & Walsh R. (1992), Phenomenology and Sequelae of 3,4-methelyenedioxumethaphetamine use. *Journal of Nervous & Mental Disease*, 180(6): 345-354.

Lee S., & McDowell, D. (1998), Drugs in Partyland: The use of drugs at a circuit party. APA national meeting, Washington DC.

Lilly, J.C. (1978), *The Scientist: a Novel Autobiography*. New York and Philadelphia: Lippincott Publishers.

Loscher W., & Honack D. (1993), Effects of the novel 5-HT1A receptor antagonist, (+)-WAY 100135 on the stereotyped behavior induced by NMDA receptor antagonist dizocilpine in rats. *European Journal of Pharmacology*, 242: 99-104.

Lammers G.J., Arends J., Deckerck A.C., Ferrari M.D., Schouwink G., & Troost J. (1993), Gammahydroxybutyrate and narcolepsy: a double blind placebo controlled study. *Sleep*, 16: 216-220.

Malhotra A.K., Pinals D.A., Weingartner H. et al. (1996), NMDA receptor function and human cognition: the effects of Ketamine in healthy volunteers. *Neuropsychopharmacology*, 14: 301-307.

McCabe E., Layne E., Sayler D., & Slusher, N. (1971), Synergy of ethanol and a natural soporific: gammahydroxybutyrate. *Science*, 171: 404-406.

McCann U.D., Ridenour A., Shaham Y., & Ricaurte G.A. (1994), Serotonin neurotoxicity after (+/−)3,4-methylenedioxymethamphetamine (MDMA; "Ecstasy"): a controlled study in humans. *Neuropsychopharmacology*, 10(2): 129-138.

McCann U., Slate S., & Ricaurte G. (1996), Adverse Reactions with 3,4-Methylendioxymehtamphetamine (MDMA: "Ecstasy"). *Drug Safety*, 15(2): 107-115.

McCann U. & Ricaurte G. (1993), Reinforcing Subjective Effects of 3,4-Methylenedioxymethamphetamine ("Ecstasy") May Be separable from its Neurotoxic Actions: Clinical Evidence. *J Clin. Psychopharmacology*, 13(3): 214-217.

McCann U. & Ricaurte G. (1991), Lasting neuropsychiatric sequelae of methylenedioxymethamphetamine ("ecstasy") in recreational users. *J Clin Psychopharmacology*, 11: 302-5.

McCann, U. & Szabo, Z. et al. (1998), Positron Emission Evidence of Toxic Effect of

MDMA (Ecstasy) on Brain Serotonin Neurons in Human Beings. *Lancet,* 352(9138):1433-7.

McDowell D. & Kleber H. (1994), MDMA, Its History and Pharmacology. *Psychiatric Annals,* 24(3): 127-130.

McDowell D. & Spitz H. (1999), *Substance Abuse: From Principles to Practice,* New York: Brunner Mazel.

McDowell D. (in press), The Treatment of Gay Men and Lesbians in Groups for Substance Abuse. In: *The APA Textbook of Group Therapy for Substance Abuse Treatment.* Washington DC: APA Press.

McKenna D., & Peroutka S. (1990), The neurochemistry and neurotoxicity of 3,4-methylenedioxymehtamphetamine, "ecstasy." *J Neurochem,* 54: 14-22.

Meyer J.S., Greifenstein F., & DeVault M. (1959), A new drug causing symptoms of sensory depravation. *J Nerv Ment Dis,* 129: 54-61.

Miller N., Gold M., & Smith D., eds. (1997), *Intoxication and Withdrawal from Marijuana, LSD, and MDMA in Manual of Therapeutics for Addictions.* New York: John Wiley and Sons.

Moretti R.J., Hassan S.Z., Goodman L.I., & Metlze H.Y. (1984), Comparison of ketamine and thiopental in health volunteers: Effects on mental status, mood, and personality. *Anest Analg,* 63: 1087-1096.

National Institute on Drug Abuse (1979), *Diagnosis and Treatment of Phencyclidine (PCP) Toxicity.* Rockville, MD: National Institute on Drug Abuse.

Newmeyer J. (1986), Some considerations on the prevalence of MDMA use. *J of Psychoactive Drugs,* 18(4): 361-362.

Newsweek (October 27, 1997), Death of the party. *Newsweek,* p. 55.

Öye N., Paulsen O., & Maurset A. (1992), Effects of ketamine on sensory perception: evidence for a role of N-Methyl D-aspartate receptors. *J Pharmacol Exp Ther,* 260: 1209-1213.

Pandit S.K., Kothary S.P., & Kumar S.M. (1980), Low dose intravenous infusion technique with ketamine. *Anesthesia,* 35: 669-675.

Pap, A. & Bradberry, C.W. (1995), Excitatory amino acid antagonists attenuate the effects of cocaine on extracellular dopamine in the nucleus accumbens. *Journal of Pharmacology and Experimental Therapeutics,* 274: 127-133.

Peroutka, S., Newman, H., & Harris, H. (1988), Subjective effects of 3,4-MDMA in Recreational Abusers. *Neuropsychopharmacology,* 11(4): 273-277.

Peroutka, S. (1990), *Ecstasy: the Clinical, Pharmacological and Neurotoxicological Effects of the drug MDMA.* Boston: Kluwer Academic Publishing.

Rattray M. (1991), Ecstasy: Towards an Understanding of the biochemical Basis of the Actions of MDMA. *Essays Biochem,* 26: 77-87.

Robinson T., Casteneda E., & Whishaw I. (1993), Effects of Cortical Serotonin Depletion Induced by 3,4-Methylenedioxymethamphetamine (MDMA) on Behavior, Before and After Additional Cholinergic Blockade. *Neuropsychopharmacology,* 8(1): 77-85.

Schifano F. (1991), Chronic atypical psychosis associated with MDMA ("ecstasy") abuse. *Lancet,* 338:1335.

Scrima L. (1992), Gamma-hydroxybutyrate (GHB) treated narcolepsy patients continue to report cataplexy controlled for up to five years. *Sleep Research,* 21: 262.

Shulgin A. (1986), The background and chemistry of MDMA. *J Psychoactive Drugs*, 18: 291-304.

Shulgin A. (1990), Chapter 1. In: *History of MDMA, in Ecstasy: the Clinical, Pharmacological and Neurotoxicological Effects of the drug MDMA* ed. Peroutka, S.: Kluwer Academic Publishing, pp. 15-68.

Siegel R.K. & Jarvik, M.E. (1975), *Drug Induced Hallucination in Animals and Man in Hallucinations*. New York: John Wiley and Sons.

Sternback H. (1991), The serotonin syndrome. *Am J Psychiatry*, 148: 705-13.

Takahara J., Yunoki S., Yakushiji W., Yamauchi J., Yamane J. & Ofuji T. (1977), Stimulatory effects of gamma-hydroxybutyric acid on growth hormone and prolactin release in humans. *J Clin Endocin Metab*, 44: 1014.

Vickers M.D. (1969), Gamma-hydroxybutyric acid. *Int Anaesthesia Clinic*, 75-89.

Watson L. & Beck J. (1986), New Age seekers: MDMA use as an adjunct to spiritual pursuit. *Journal of Psychoactive Drugs*, 23(3): 261-270.

SPECIAL POPULATIONS AND TREATMENT SETTINGS

Treating Gay, Lesbian, Bisexual and Transgender Professionals with Addictive Disease

Penelope P. Ziegler, MD

SUMMARY. This article explores the complexities of treating profession-als who are addicted and who are also gay, lesbian, bisexual or transgend-ered. It provides an overview of the special needs of this population, fo-cusing on denial issues, defenses and resistance. In addition, it offers detailed case examples which illustrate specific complications, including medical and psychiatric co-morbidity, internalized and societal homopho-bia, codependency, return to practice and monitoring issues, and chal-lenges encountered by gay, lesbian, bisexual and transgender persons par-ticipating in Twelve-Step programs. Emphasis is placed on the most effective approaches for providing training and ongoing supervision for addiction treatment professionals working with these patients. *[Article copies available for a fee from The Haworth Document Delivery Service: 1-800-342-9678. E-mail address: <getinfo@haworthpressinc.com> Website: <http://www.HaworthPress.com>]*

KEYWORDS. Homosexuality, alcoholism, addiction, gay alcoholics, gay addicts, impaired professionals, homophobia, addicted physicians, gay professionals

Dr. Penelope P. Ziegler is affiliated with the William J. Farley Center, 5477 Mooretown Road, Williamsburg, VA 23188.

[Haworth co-indexing entry note]: "Treating Gay, Lesbian, Bisexual and Transgender Professionals with Addictive Disease." Ziegler, Penelope P. Co-published simultaneously in *Journal of Gay & Lesbian Psychotherapy* (The Haworth Medical Press, an imprint of The Haworth Press, Inc.) Vol. 3, No. 3/4, 2000, pp. 59-68; and: *Addictions in the Gay and Lesbian Community* (ed: Jeffrey R. Guss, and Jack Drescher) The Haworth Medical Press, an imprint of The Haworth Press, Inc., 2000, pp. 59-68. Single or multiple copies of this article are available from The Haworth Document Delivery Service [1-800-342-9678, 9:00 a.m. - 5:00 p.m. (EST). E-mail address: getinfo@haworthpressinc.com].

© 2000 by The Haworth Press, Inc. All rights reserved.

Professionals requiring treatment for chemical dependency present special challenges to the treatment provider. In general, their defenses are highly sophisticated and intellectualized, and are reinforced by social stereotypes and extreme definitions of who is an addict, who is an alcoholic. Additional complications arise when the patient is also gay, lesbian, bisexual and/or transgender. Many persons who are both professionals and members of a sexual minority may emerge from traditional addiction treatment settings without the reduction of denial and acceptance of the need for continued treatment of their chronic disease. Without this acceptance, there is a greater risk of relapse to active addiction or substitution of alternative dependencies.

Certain defenses and denial strategies are typical and predictable, depending on the patient's professional identity. Health care professionals, such as physicians, nurses, dentists and pharmacists, tend to rely on minimization ("I'm working every day, I'm receiving more referrals than ever, I've never had a malpractice suit, lost a job, etc."), rationalization ("I needed those pills for my migraine headaches, insomnia, anxiety, etc."), and comparison ("All the surgical residents drink as much as I do, so if I'm an alcoholic. . . ."). Lawyers also minimize and compare; in addition, they tend to take the adversarial role with treaters, focusing on details at the expense of the larger picture. Those in the arts express the belief that chemicals are essential to their creativity, and that without drugs they would be unable to be spontaneous and to overcome performance anxiety. Scientists and engineers may critique the addiction literature or become highly knowledgeable about treatment and recovery while never connecting with themselves or others on an emotional level. This approach may result in periods of abstinence with no accompanying improvement in stress management skills, followed by relapse.

In general, since professionals are accustomed to having and wielding power, grasping the concept of powerlessness over their addictions is extremely threatening. Most individuals who have achieved success in a professional endeavor have depended on personality traits such as self-reliance, determination and persistence. This can make bonding with a mutual help support system difficult and even threatening to many.

An additional area of complexity for many professionals entering treatment involves special relapse risks that must be addressed prior to the individual's return to work. Health care professionals who have become addicted to chemicals that will be readily available in the workplace and that they may be required to handle as a part of their daily job requirements will be at very high risk of relapse on the job. Attorneys will need to explore the issue of the alcohol-centered power lunch, the firm's expectations for entertaining clients and the appropriate response to the offer of a drink by the senior partner. The rock guitarist will need to deal with his band members' heroin use, the painter with her perceived inability to create without marijuana, the actor with his stage fright requiring Klonopin. Some professionals will also be facing licensure issues, discrimination in continued employment and other consequences requiring effective advocacy and possible ongoing monitoring. Confidentiality and protection of privacy are essential for all patients, but may present special challenges when the patient is a high-profile professional.

When the professional in treatment is also gay, lesbian, bisexual and/or transgender, an additional set of potential needs comes into play. Assessment of this patient must include exploration of his or her level of self-acceptance as a gay, lesbian, bisexual or transgendered person. This may be viewed as falling on a continuum from severe internalized homophobia with denial of sexual orientation and/or gender identity, through shame-based "double life" adaptations, through varying degrees of "outness" which may or may not include professional peer support systems. Irrespective of the individual's internal level of comfort, some professions demand total secrecy from their GLBT practitioners, while in other professions, certain specific types of work require extreme discretion. A professional faces special problems when he or she is planning a change in gender identification, and needs to anticipate the reactions of others.

Some case examples, which represent patients evaluated and/or treated in a specialized partial hospital treatment program for addicted professionals (with altered details intended to protect the privacy of the individuals), will illustrate the complexity of these cases and the need for highly individualized treatment planning.

Case Example #1: A 38 year old Caucasian male registered nurse, Mr. G., was referred to the treatment center because of dependence on parenteral meperidine and morphine, which he had been diverting from his job in the Medical Intensive Care Unit of a large teaching hospital. Despite six years of previously outstanding service, he had been terminated from his job and reported to the Nursing Board, which had suspended his license. The patient had a long history of heavy social alcohol and marijuana use dating to adolescence, when he began going to gay bars. He started injecting drugs three years ago when his partner of four years died of AIDS-related lymphoma. At that time he was seronegative but had since participated in unprotected receptive anal intercourse with three different men and had not been HIV tested regularly. He had been severely depressed and had had suicidal fantasies continuously since his partner's death, but had not made a direct attempt or plan. However, he viewed his sexual behavior as "slow suicide." He had no history of prior substance abuse treatment or psychiatric treatment. He was estranged from his parents, who had not been able to accept his sexual orientation, but had a close relationship with his sister, who was three years older and married to an alcoholic man. His father had drunk heavily and was physically abusive to him, his sister and his mother throughout his childhood; however, the father had stopped drinking 10 years ago after a religious conversion.

The patient was diagnosed with polysubstance dependence (opioid, alcohol and cannabis), with unresolved grief issues and a possible depressive disorder. A treatment plan was implemented as follows:

1. Mr. G. was safely detoxified and medically stabilized. HIV testing revealed that he was HIV positive with significant viral load and adequate CD4 counts. He was evaluated by a family physician experienced in HIV/AIDS treatment and started on a multi-drug regimen. He received extensive pre- and post-test counseling.

2. Following detoxification, depression was an obvious issue, and was approached with a combination of antidepressant medication and behavioral-cognitive individual therapy, in addition to addiction-focused group therapy. Also, the patient was referred to support groups for newly diagnosed HIV-positive patients, and for surviving partners of men who had died from AIDS.

3. The patient's sister was invited to attend the family program, and also did conjoint work with the patient, exploring their childhood experiences in their abusive alcoholic family. Both began attending Adult Children of Alcoholics meetings.

4. Mr. G. was encouraged to enroll in the Nursing Board's monitoring program, and was able to have his license re-instated on a probationary status after completing the primary treatment program and receiving advocacy from the program's medical director. He agreed to take naltrexone and to work in a setting where he would not be administering controlled drugs for at least six months.

5. Mr. G. attended general and gay-specific Twelve Step meetings, as well as a Twelve-Step support group for recovering nurses.

Case Example #2: A 32 year old Caucasian lesbian physician, Dr. P., was referred for evaluation after she was confronted by the Physician Health Committee about self-prescribing Fioricet with codeine and Stadol nasal spray for her migraine headaches. Although she was under the care of a neurologist and had a treatment protocol which included both preventive and abortive strategies for the headaches, it was clear from her own report and the pharmacy records that she was totally unable to comply with the protocol. She was using 4-5 times the recommended amounts of Stadol plus very large dosages of barbiturates and codeine, unknown to the treating neurologist. The patient had a history of classic migraine dating to age 14, but with marked increase in frequency and severity of headaches over the past two years, corresponding in time to her first committed relationship with a woman. Dr.

P. was very fearful about her family learning of her relationship and was convinced that they would disown her. She and her partner argued about this frequently, with the partner encouraging her to be more socially active in the lesbian community. The patient stated that she had been aware of her orientation since about age 17, but had been ashamed of it and had had several very unsatisfying relationships with men, including an engagement she broke off weeks before the wedding. She had had only brief sexual encounters with women prior to meeting her current partner. She viewed her homosexuality as a sign of "deep psychological problems." She gave a history of having been sexually molested from age six to ten by a paternal uncle. She had always seen this as the "cause" of her homosexuality. There was a strongly positive family history of alcoholism.

A treatment plan was developed to address the patient's complicated addiction, psychiatric and medical issues.

1. Dr. P. required a medically monitored detoxification from barbiturates and opiates. After completing detoxification, during which she had severe rebound headaches, she worked with the team to develop a headache management protocol which included preventive medication, use of a triptan preparation for abortive therapy, complementary therapies including relaxation training, acupuncture and massage. Headache frequency and severity decreased dramatically over the next few months.

2. Intensive individual and couples work focused on acceptance of sexual orientation, improved self-esteem and identification and expression of emotions, especially anger. Dr. P. was able to recognize that her orientation was not indicative of underlying psychopathology, but was a normal variant unrelated to her history of sexual abuse. The abuse history *had* resulted in serious trust issues, communication problems and other relationship difficulties. The patient and her partner were taught techniques for direct communication and assertiveness. Some exploration of the sexual trauma was begun, and EMDR techniques were utilized with positive results.

3. Dr. P. chose a Twelve-Step sponsor who was an older lesbian with long-term recovery, and practiced the difficult behavior of calling her sponsor daily, asking for support and direction, and following suggestions and recommendations. She made excellent progress in modifying her previous "help-rejecting complainer" behavior.

Case Example #3: A 29 year old African-American gay male second-year anesthesiology resident, Dr. S., was referred for detoxification and addiction treatment after it was discovered by his residency director that he was using large amounts of fentanyl and sufentanyl intravenously. The patient had a long history of polysubstance dependence dating to age 12, and most recently including, in addition to the anesthetic agents, current use of cocaine, XTC, GHB, Ketamine ("Special K") and amyl nitrate. He had been participating in unsafe sex with multiple partners in the context of his involvement in the "Rave" scene and attendance at circuit parties. He was estranged from his family and denied any feelings of loss in this context, while refusing to discuss his family history of addiction or other psychiatric illness. He described his childhood as "a hell best forgotten." In group therapy, he was hostile and provocative. Peers complained that he was verbally threatening and refused to participate in community activities.

1. This patient had extreme trust problems and required much patience and compassion on the part of the therapist, who received intensive supervision while working with this individual. Dr. S. responded to some degree to a mood stabilizer and antidepressant medication. He continued to test limits, to act out and to have episodes of intense anger. A behavioral contract was useful.
2. Major childhood trauma issues were suspected and hinted at by the patient. Dr. S. began individual therapy with a specialist in Post-Traumatic Stress Disorder, with whom he could continue to work in long term therapy.
3. Despite his efforts to alienate his peer group, Dr. S. was accepted and supported by peers and by the recovering community in the area. Sexual compulsivity was identified as a component of his addiction, and he attended a gay group of Sex and Love Addicts Anonymous (SLAA) in addition to his AA and NA meeting. Attempts to work with a gay male sponsor were not successful due to the sexual tension and seductive behavior demonstrated by the patient. He worked more effectively with an African-American female sponsor, with whom he was able to form a somewhat trusting alliance.
4. Despite initial resistance and anger, Dr. S. eventually was able to accept the need to redirect his career plans toward a safer specialty. After demonstrating an ability to remain abstinent and cooperate with the state medical society's monitoring program for a period of six months, he began a residency in Family Medicine.

Case Example #4: A 46 year old male to female preoperative transsexual surgeon, Dr. A., had self-referred for treatment after hospital privileges were suspended. Dr. A., who had been in practice in this suburban community for 15 years as a male, had come to work on numerous occasions with alcohol on the breath. Operating room personnel were very disturbed, because Dr. A. had begun dressing as a woman, requesting to use the female locker room, and asking colleagues and staff to use a new feminine name. The hospital medical staff office, while attempting to be sensitive to the physician's needs, was at a total loss as to how to deal with the situation. Dr. A. had been seeing a therapist for several years. In addition to the gender identity issues, Dr. A. had been diagnosed as alcohol-dependent, with the recommendation to attend Alcoholics Anonymous. However, a consulting psychiatrist was prescribing Klonopin and Ambien for generalized anxiety and insomnia. Dr. A. had been unable to sustain more than two weeks of continuous abstinence from alcohol, and was unwilling to attend A.A. meetings near home. Dr. A's estranged wife was refusing to allow visitation with their two children, citing "sexual perversion" as a risk to the children's mental health.

1. After detoxification from alcohol, it became clear that Dr. A was experiencing hypomanic symptoms which responded well to Depakote. She participated in the treatment program in her new identity as a female. Treatment team members required frequent opportunities to express their reactions to the situation and to explore their intolerance and bias. Gradually they were able to achieve an acceptance of the patient's gender identity.

2. After her mood stabilized, Dr. A. was able to understand the impossibility of successfully making a gender identity change "in situ" in her home community. She worked with the medical directors of two physician peer support programs to locate a new practice opportunity in a community that had no preconceived images and expectations. Twelve Step meetings and other support systems in the new community came to know her as a recovering woman.

3. After several months of recovery, Dr. A began having supervised visits with her children, who continued to struggle with the profound changes this had brought to their world. The children had begun receiving individual therapy and participating in a support group for children whose parents are divorcing; they resisted attending Al-ateen.

Case Example #5: A 45 year old Latina pediatrician was referred for evaluation after an incident of bizarre behavior at the hospital with a urine drug screen positive for codeine and alcohol. Dr. F. was married to a family physician and had four children under age 12. She also had a long term intimate relationship with Martina, a nursing assistant in her office, with whom she often spent weekends and vacations. She described herself as bisexual, and expressed a determination to continue both relationships, stating that she loved both partners equally. She reported a regular pattern of drinking two or three glasses of wine each evening after work, and her husband confirmed this pattern. Two days prior to the incident at the hospital, she had sustained a severe ankle sprain in a bicycle accident and had been prescribed Tylenol #3 by the orthopedic surgeon who had evaluated the ankle. The evening of the incident, she was on call. She had taken two

Tylenol #3 tablets and had two glasses of wine after dinner, and then been called into the ER. While evaluating a child who had been injured in a motor vehicle crash, she had been verbally insulting and abusive to the child's mother. When nurses attempted to intervene, they described Dr. F. as belligerent and seeming to be intoxicated. Dr. F. believed that her husband and children were not aware of the relationship with Martina. However, during the evaluation it became clear that the "secret" was not only known to all but was a focus of severely dysfunctional, triangulated relationships among the children and husband, and between Martina and two of the children. Dr. F.'s affect was depressed and anxious, and she acknowledged feeling desperate and overwhelmed by her efforts to juggle her relationships, professional activities and mothering responsibilities.

Dr. F. did not meet the diagnostic criteria for substance dependence. However, she had demonstrated very poor judgement by drinking alcohol while on call, and by combining alcohol and opiates. She agreed to sign a contract for abstinence from alcohol and other drugs not prescribed for her by an attending physician, and for a one-year random urine drug-monitoring program.

1. A depressive disorder was present, and recommendation was made for ongoing outpatient psychiatric care and a trial of antidepressant medication. (Medication has not brought about a dramatic change in affect or anxiety level.)
2. The patient began seeing a therapist who is experienced in working with complex and entangled relationship issues. As she developed a beginning trust in the therapist, she started to explore her dysfunctional family of origin, including the mixed messages received from her parents about intimacy and commitment, and possible sexual abuse. She was not ready to engage in any conjoint work with her husband, children or lover.

Each of these cases presents a complicated, multifaceted and multi-diagnostic challenge to an evaluation and/or treatment team. Chemical dependency education and group therapy focused on denial reduction and self-diagnosis of addiction will be essential in each case, but treatment planning will also need to include interventions focused on the complex psychosocial factors involved. Although no reliable data are available, reports from gay, lesbian, bisexual and transgender patients who have had previous addiction treatment indicate that most treatment programs are not prepared to deal effectively with such cases. Very few treatment facilities and outpatient programs provide inservice training for treatment professionals (physicians, counselors, nurses, activity therapists, etc.) geared toward improving competence in working with GLBT patients. While overt homophobia may be unusual, heterosexist assumptions and attitudes discourage self-disclosure and open discussion of orientation and gender identity issues. Many patients report that, during previous treatment experiences, they were not even asked about sexual orientation, or felt that they could not rely on the counselor or physician to protect their privacy. The presumption of heterosexuality is even stronger when a professional presents for treatment.

Only a sensitized and culturally competent treatment team, in which members have been encouraged to explore their own issues with homophobia and heterosexism, can approach these challenging cases and develop an individualized treatment approach to address all relevant issues. Treatment providers also need to function as advocates for these patients as they re-enter professional practice. This may involve educating employers, practice partners, hospital administrators, etc.; assisting the patient in finding a sensitive, accepting work environment; dealing with licensing boards, disciplinary systems and/or legal entities; working with family members to overcome the "double stigma" phenomenon; making appropriate referrals for ongoing therapy, medical management, psychiatric treatment, and relationship counseling; helping the patient locate support systems and deal with often insensitive but required profession-specific monitoring groups. The physician or other treatment provider is attempting to achieve a difficult balance between sensitivity to the patient's individual need and reinforcing the patient's sense of uniqueness and separateness, which can undermine recovery.

Addiction psychiatrists and other physicians are in a position to improve the quality of treatment available to GLBT professionals with addictive disorders by promoting increased awareness of the issues and requesting and developing inservice training programs for addiction professionals which are geared toward improved competence in treating this special population. Effective and sensitive treatment can be provided either in a specialized GLBT addiction treatment setting or in a mainstream program, but only if the providers have received adequate training and supervision in evaluation, treatment planning, meeting professional re-entry challenges, and providing monitoring and advocacy.

REFERENCES

Bissell, L. & Haberman, P. (1984), *Alcoholism in the Professions.* New York: Oxford University Press.

Bissell, L. & Crosby, L. (1989), *To Care Enough: Intervention with Chemically Dependent Colleagues.* Minneapolis: Johnson Institute Books.

Centrella, M. (1994), Physician addiction and impairment–current thinking: a review. *J Addic Dis* 13:91-105.

Finnegan, D. & McNally, E. (1987), *Dual Identities: Counseling Chemically Dependent Gay Men and Lesbians.* Center City, MN: Hazelden.

Hedberg, H., Ziegler, P., Mansky, P. (1997), Physician chemical dependency: trends, issues, treatment and consequences. *Med Prac Manage,* 1:186-190.

Kettlehack, G. (1999), *Vastley More Than That: Stories of Lesbians and Gay Men In Recovery*. Center City, MN: Hazelden.

Millige, C., Young, M. (1990), Perceived acceptance and social isolation among recovering homosexual alcoholics. *Int J Addict* 25:947-955.

Weinstein, D., ed. (1992), *Lesbians and Gay Men: Chemical Dependency Treatment Issues*. Binghamton. NY: Harrington Park Press.

Ziebold, T. & Mongeon, J. (1985), *Gay and Sober: Directions for Counseling and Therapy*. Binghamton. NY: Harrington Park Press.

Ziegler, P. (1992), Monitoring impaired physicians: a tool for relapse prevention. *PA Med*, 95:38-40.

Gay Teens and Substance Use Disorders: Assessment and Treatment

Eva D. Olson, MD

SUMMARY. Substance use is very common among adolescents with as many as 50% reporting use of illicit substances and 80% reporting use of alcohol by their senior year of high school. Gay and lesbian teens are reported to be at greater risk for substance use. Stress mediates this increased risk due to the contradiction of needing to establish an integrated sense of self, while doing so runs the risk of peer and family rejection, fears for personal safety, and the ongoing experience of homophobic remarks and jokes that are common in today's high schools. Assessment for substance abuse in adolescents needs to be comprehensive, documenting a patient's sexual history, his or her stage in the coming out process, and issues of safety at home, school and the community. Gay-sensitive treatment planning can facilitate greater treatment compliance and abstinence. *[Article copies available for a fee from The Haworth Document Delivery Service: 1-800-342-9678. E-mail address: <getinfo@haworthpressinc.com> Website: <http://www.HaworthPress.com>]*

KEYWORDS. Homosexuality, adolescence, substance abuse, assessment, treatment

Adolescent substance use represents a significant public health problem due to its high prevalence and multiple adverse consequences. Recent reports reveal that nearly a quarter (22%) of all eighth graders had tried marijuana

Dr. Eva D. Olson is Clinical Assistant Professor, Department of Psychiatry, University of Michigan, Ann Arbor, MI 48109.

[Haworth co-indexing entry note]: "Gay Teens and Substance Use Disorders: Assessment and Treatment." Olson, Eva D. Co-published simultaneously in *Journal of Gay & Lesbian Psychotherapy* (The Haworth Medical Press, an imprint of The Haworth Press, Inc.) Vol. 3, No. 3/4, 2000, pp. 69-80; and: *Addictions in the Gay and Lesbian Community* (ed: Jeffrey R. Guss, and Jack Drescher) The Haworth Medical Press, an imprint of The Haworth Press, Inc., 2000, pp. 69-80. Single or multiple copies of this article are available from The Haworth Document Delivery Service [1-800-342-9678, 9:00 a.m. - 5:00 p.m. (EST). E-mail address: getinfo@haworthpressinc.com].

© 2000 by The Haworth Press, Inc. All rights reserved.

and almost half (49%) of all twelfth graders had said they had done so. The statistics for alcohol use in the past month are similar: 24% of eighth graders and 52% of twelfth graders (Johnston, 1998). Johnston and his colleagues have associated high levels of substance use with two main factors; a decreased perception of harm or dangerousness of use, and a high perception of acceptability in their peer group.

The prevalence of alcohol use disorders in a cohort of adolescents, 14-16 years old, range from three to four percent (Cohen et al., 1993) to almost a third (32%) of a cohort of high-school seniors (Reinhertz et al., 1993). Fulkerson and colleagues (1999) recently reported on a large population-based adolescent sample of 78,800 14-18 year old high school students. They found 18,803 (25%) of the youth reported substance use and met diagnostic criteria for at least one substance use disorder during the previous 12 months.

There are multiple risk factors associated with substance experimentation leading to a substance use disorder. The most frequently noted is the presence of substance use disorders within the family setting. This likely represents both genetic factors and an associated decrease in parental monitoring or supervision which leads to a decrease in parental control of behavior. Personality factors, such as impulsivity, anxiousness, alienation, poor self-esteem and low conformity all have been linked with increased risk for substance abuse and dependence. Temperamental factors such as novelty seeking, and stress and trauma have also been associated with increased substance use disorders (Dawes, 1999; DeBord et al., 1998).

SUBSTANCE USE AND GLB TEENS

While substance use among adolescents is reported at alarming rates, two studies have found that substance abuse and dependence is even more prevalent in samples of gay and lesbian youth (Remafedi, 1987, 1991; Garofalo, 1998). One recent study (Lock and Steiner, 1999), however, did not report an increased risk of this population. It should be noted that Remafedi's study recruited their subjects from gay support groups, drop-in centers, bars and acquaintance referrals which may skew the data in favor of finding an association. Garofalo's study was community based with 3,365 subjects. One hundred and twenty-nine (3.8%) identified themselves as gay, lesbian, bisexual or not sure. His findings suggest that homosexuality increased the risk for health problems, suicidality, victimization, sexual risk taking and use of multiple substances. Lock and Steiner's study of 106 (5.9%) self-identified gay, lesbian and bisexual youth were drawn from a large community sample of 1,769 12-18 year olds. The instrument they used encompassed five domains: General Risk Taking (drug use, running away, alcohol use and reckless driving), Mental Health Problems, Sexual Victimization and Risk, Eating and Dietary Problems, and General Health Problems. They found increased mental heath risk, sexual risk taking and general health risk but not in the general risk taking domain where the probe for alcohol and drug use lay. In reports of substance abuse among gay and lesbian adults, the incidence of substance abuse is estimated to be 28-35% (Cabaj, 1996).

There are many possible contributory factors to an association of increased risk of substance use disorder among gay and lesbian teens. Common to all these is increased stress. Self-identification as a gay or lesbian is an extraordinarily long and stressful process. Doing so as a teenager is a terrifying experience. Fears of family and peer rejection are very potent. As a gay or lesbian adolescent, fears for one's physical safety at home, in the community and at school are very real (Remafedi, 1987; D'Augelli, 1998). In addition to issues of personal rejection and safety, the homophobic remarks and jokes that are regularly tolerated in schools and homes conflict with the primary task of adolescence, that of establishing a healthy, coherent sense of self. A gay or lesbian teenager incorporates these negative attitudes and experiences as he or she navigates adolescence. The result is that homophobia may be internalized and acted out.

Coping with these stresses takes many forms which are then influenced by the age of the teen. The developing teen is evolving cognitively, socially, emotionally and physically. The parents of the teen must evolve and support the teen's need for separation, individuation, and autonomy and yet remain available and interested emotionally. Within this context, same sex attraction begins to emerge around eleven years old (D'Agelli and Hershberger, 1993; Herdt and Boxer, 1993). The early teen is still highly dependent and relatively concrete cognitively such that dealing with the concurrent social pressure for heterosexuality is overwhelming. Common early defenses to these conflicts are denial, repression of any sexuality, or compulsive or exaggerated heterosexuality. These reactions contribute to the isolation young gays and lesbians feel. In addition, when one is not safe to explore his or her identity, but instead feels pressure to hide, there may develop a true-false dichotomy of self. The stress of vigilant hiding often leads to anxiety and depression.

Substance use can emerge both in the context of self medication, and in relation to self marginalization. Moving out of the mainstream world to a place where there is greater tolerance for a wider range of behavior affords the teen room to explore gendered and sexual behaviors, but may prematurely foreclose experimentation in other areas of life, be it sports, leadership opportunities, etc. Substance use may well assuage the extreme cognitive and emotional conflicts created in establishing a public or false self. It is not uncommon for a gay or lesbian's first same-sex sexual experience to occur while high or intoxicated. It is likely the substance use decreases inhibitions, denial, anxiety, or even fear of gay sex.

As gay and lesbian teens develop, they gradually become less frightened and more accepting of their attractions and fantasies. This frequently leads to self-labeling as gay or lesbian. Two studies indicated the average age of this self recognition to be 15 years old (D'Agelli and Hershberger, 1993; Herdt and Boxer, 1993). This can be a freeing experience as it can allow teens to rework their self definition with more accurate information and allow for a more conscious exploration of themselves within the world. However, more complex and potentially destructive emotions may also emerge. The anxiety of hiding and passing as a heterosexual often continues yet may well be transformed into anger at having to hide and pass for protection from violence, verbal (55%) and physical (30%), negative reaction from peers (41%) and a strong negative reaction from parents (43%) (Remafedi, 1987). The anxiety also has a new dimension, that of anticipation/terror in knowing their desire to meet other gays, preferably teens, and then planning and succeeding in that venture. In the last decade, this has been made somewhat easier in some communities with the establishment of gay, lesbian and bisexual community centers, gay youth support groups, and gay-straight alliances in some high schools. However, the fear of being caught in this exploration remains enormous and only a minority of teens are able to overcome such fear and seek support. The average age of the first disclosure to another person of one's homosexual identity is 16 years old (D'Agelli and Hershberger, 1993; Herdt and Boxer, 1993).

The interplay of social isolation with feelings of anxiety, anger, and fear may lead to depression, chronic stress and a sense of overwhelming helplessness. These symptoms are also commonly identified as risk factors in substance abusing teens.

ASSESSMENT

When working with teenagers, whether it is from a substance abuse frame of reference or a mental health perspective, the assessment of a teen needs to include a broad range of inquiry. The first step is to establish the ground rules. The teen should be told how the information elicited during the assessment process will be used and with whom it will be shared. He or she should be assured that confidentiality will be maintained unless the teen is engaged in behaviors that are injurious or life-threatening to self or others. Honesty is to be promoted and secrets avoided lest there be collusion to undermine the treatment. The clinician should then begin to establish rapport with the teen and the parents. To do this, I begin by meeting with the teen and the adults who accompanied him or her to the assessment. I ask the teenager what they were told about the purpose of the visit. Sometimes there is a shared understanding of that purpose; other times, the evaluation must begin by clarifying discrepancies. Once we all have a shared understanding of the task and issues of confidentiality have been clarified, meeting with the adolescent alone is recommended. Meeting alone with the teen communicates respect for their emerging individuality and autonomy, and an interest in their life story. Listening without assumptions or quick judgements is important to establishing rapport. The same can also be said for interactions with the parents. Whether a mental health or substance abuse assessment is being done, a clinician may have the feeling that he or she is hearing the stories of two different people, instead of the tale of only one teenager. Clinicians need to be careful not to pick "sides" because each story has elements of truth. To do a complete assessment one must listen to the "music" of the stories. A clinician must ask: Does each story make sense? Does each hang together as a whole or are there missing pieces? Do the facts support the narrative? Is the emotional tune consistent with the words/narrative? A clinician's task is to listen at multiple levels, develop a sense of what is missing and then develop hypotheses as to how the teen's problems evolved. Ideally, the hypotheses motivate the treatment choices and structure.

The specifics of a substance abuse assessment are well described in many texts (Kaminer, 1994; Graham and Schultz, 1998; SAMHSA, 1993). The problem with what is described in the texts is twofold. First, some assessments completely leave out evaluating a teenager's sexuality and identity formation (Kaminer, 1994). In my view, adolescents are sexual beings even if they are not sexually active. This is an important part of their identity and to neglect it is to neglect an important aspect of the teen. As noted above, becoming aware of one's homoerotic feelings is extraordinarily stressful. It is therefore essential to include evaluation of sexual identity in any substance abuse assessment. Second, though the need for sexual identity assessment is noted briefly in the American Society of Addiction Medicine (1998) and SAMHSA (1993), the bulk of substance abuse research literature fails to include sexual orientation either as a piece of demographic data or as a factor when probing or assessing risk for substance abuse. By failing to do so, we acquire no information as to whether homosexuality itself is a risk factor. The stress of socio-cultural stigma, homophobia and violence are the associated risk factors including the teen's participation in the substance use culture within the gay and lesbian community where bars are core meeting places promoting substance abuse.

The elements of a substance abuse assessment include a comprehensive substance use history (Table 1); medical history, including history prior to substance use onset, injuries, and illnesses; a complete physical exam including assessment for withdrawal potential and labs (Table 2); complete psychiatric assessment (Table 3); and social history (Table 4) which would probe for areas where life functioning is impaired. Examples of questions for the sexual history are demonstrated in Table 5.

There are multiple tools available to guide the assessment process. These

TABLE 1. Substance Abuse History

For each substance obtain the following:

- Age at first use, length of time to second use
- Pattern of use: amount, frequency, fluctuation (max, abstinence), setting, route
- Means of acquiring the substance
- Effect–psychological and physiological, during and after use, positive and negative
- Tolerance, withdrawal, blackouts
- Behaviors when high
- Identify what triggers use, assess relapse potential
- Treatment history, attitude toward treatment

TABLE 2. Physical Exam and Labs

- Assess potential for withdrawal: blood pressure, heart rate, respiratory rate
- Electrolytes, calcium, magnesium
- Liver function tests: SGOT, SGPT, GGTP
- Complete blood count
- Urine toxicology
- Breathalyzer
- Blood toxicology

TABLE 3. Psychiatric History

- ADHD
- Mood disorders, depression and bipolar disorder
- Suicidal thoughts, suicidal behaviors, para-suicidal behaviors
- Anxiety disorders
- Post Traumatic Stress Disorder
- Eating disorders
- Conduct disorder and anti-social behaviors
- Risk taking behaviors

TABLE 4. Social History (Assess for Impairment in Life Function)

- Family system, relationships
- Peer relationships, romantic relationships
- School performance, adjustment, coping
- Work history, chores (how do they get money?)
- Leisure, recreation, hobbies–past and current
- Legal–past and current, or illegal activity but not caught
- Sexuality–first activity (wanted, unwanted, mixed), risk taking, trauma, sexual orientation
- History of any trauma
- Religious beliefs–past and current

TABLE 5. Sexual History

- Have you begun to notice or be aware of romantic or sexual interests in boys, girls or both?
- When you watch TV or go to the movies, do you find yourself attracted to men, women or both?
- When you are at school, at the mall or walking down the street, do you find yourself noticing or being attracted to guys, girls or both equally?
- Do you masturbate? When you masturbate, do you think about or create a picture of guys or girls mostly?
- Have you ever gone out with a guy or a girl?
- How far have you gone with a guy or girl?
- If they have had intercourse, have they had anal intercourse?
- Have they ever felt coerced or forced to do something sexually that they didn't really want to do?
- Have they done anything sexually that they later regretted or wish they hadn't done?

include screening instruments such as the CAGE, AUDIT, MAST, DAST and the PESQ, which probe only for substance use and some adverse sequelae, though not risk factors. There are assessment instruments (e.g., DUSI, POS-IT) which are designed to obtain detailed substance use history, and survey functioning and impairment in several domains. Semi-structured and structured diagnostic tools such as the DISC-R, K-SADS-E, are solely for DSM-IV diagnoses. Regardless of how the assessment process is assembled, the key remains to keep the teen and his or her family central within the process. Doing so requires that the facts and information obtained with any tool be integrated with the history and interview of the teen and then again with the history from the parents. It is this integration which allows for individualized treatment planning.

TREATMENT

Once the assessment is completed, feedback and recommendations are given to the adolescent and parents or guardians. Feedback given in a thoughtful manner accomplishes many tasks. It enhances the treatment alliance, increases motivation to comply with recommendations, recognizes the adolescent's needs for autonomy, recognizes the parent's need for inclusion in the treatment and it is developmentally sensitive. When addressing a teenager, the feedback should link substance use consequences to the substance use using the teen's own words and examples. Next, the clinician shows how the teen is not meeting his or her goals due to consequences related to substance use. The treatment recommendation should then facilitate the teen to meet his/her own goal(s). Throughout this process, the clinician actively avoids conflict and can cope with the resistance encountered. Examples of this include techniques such as, frequent clarification of what the teen or parent is saying, avoiding assumptions of what's on their mind and what they are feeling. Avoid reacting to defensive behavior with confrontation, but do keep in mind the common underlying feelings of vulnerability and inadequacy. Humor is always a good tool with teens and parents, too. Keeping the parents in the loop with information, education and guidance helps build and keep a treatment alliance with them.

In our treatment center, a common tool for demonstrating respect for the emerging autonomy of the teen involves the negotiation of a behavioral or "home" contract with rewards and consequences. Such a contract usually includes increases and decreases in independence, respectively. The success or failure of the contract is controlled by the teenager's behavior. Parents usually need guidance in how to create enough space (e.g., not nagging or reminding) for their teen to succeed or fail on his or her own. The contract itself is a written document reflecting communication between the teen and parents about specific behaviors and the natural and logical consequences of failure to meet the behavioral guidelines. See Appendix 1 and 2 for examples.

Creating a treatment plan for the gay or lesbian teen poses some unique challenges. First consideration is the type of program to recommend. An ideal program is one that is gay-affirming. Cabaj (1996) suggests that self-acceptance of one's homosexuality is "crucial" to recovery from substance abuse. However, a program that is open about accepting a range of sexualities may be too threatening to a teen who is just beginning to self identify as gay or lesbian or may inhibit parents from being supportive of treatment. On the other hand, outside of urban centers, many communities may have only one teen substance abuse program to chose from and it may or may not be gay sensitive. Due to these issues, the following may help guide treatment planning. Did the assessment indicate a link between the substance abuse and stress of being gay or lesbian? If so, then an individual treatment may be more appropriate to allow a safe place to directly explore these issues. If not, group therapy should be considered, but safety within the group would need to be assessed so the teen would be safe from homophobic remarks and victimization. There is no clear type of treatment, CBT or interpersonal (Myers et al., 1996, Kaminer and Burleson, 1999), that has shown to be better than another. Teenagers generally tend to do well in a group because they respect and tolerate confrontation by peers.

Gay AA/NA groups should be considered but may not be appropriate for younger gay teens for two reasons. First, these groups tend to be for adults, hence are not developmentally appropriate, yet can be supportive in terms of sexual orientation and sobriety. Second, younger teens are more dependent on parents for transportation, and if the teen's parents are not aware of the sexual orientation issues, then the secrecy and stress of exposure are likely relapse triggers. Teen AA/NA meetings should generally be a part of the treatment plan. However, the clinician needs to monitor for homophobia within that may compromise the teen's treatment.

Family work is almost always indicated when working with substance abusing teens. Here again, the clinician needs to be mindful of the subject of sexuality accidentally becoming an issue without prior preparation between the patient and clinician. I usually meet with the parents without the teen present for several sessions, assessing the parent's understanding of the developmental needs of their teenager, stage of sexual development, and the parent's emotional tolerance for their child's need to begin to establish independence, autonomy and a separate identity. Once I have an understanding of the parent's awareness of and tolerance for normal developmental issues, then I can better assist the teenager in developing realistic coping strategies regarding stresses related to their sexual orientation.

CONCLUSION

Substance use and substance use disorders are unfortunately common problems amongst teenagers. There is also a growing body of literature suggesting that gay and lesbian teens are at greater risk for such problems. The stress of being or emerging as gay or lesbian is suggested as a significant mediating factor for this association. Due to this linkage, a thorough assessment, which by definition includes a complete sexual history is essential for any treatment plan to be truly effective. Treatment planning that is both gay and teen sensitive enhances the establishment of a positive treatment alliance and therefore treatment compliance and abstinence.

REFERENCES

Cabaj, R (1996), Substance Abuse in Gay Men, Lesbians, and Bisexuals. In *Textbook of Homosexuality and Mental Health*. (Cabaj, R. & Stein, T., Eds.), Washington DC: American Psychiatric Press, Inc., pp. 783-799.

Cohen, P, Cohen, J, Kasen, S, Velez, CN, Hartmark, C, Johnson, J, Rojas, M, Brook, J, Streuning, EL (1993), An epidemiological study of disorders in late childhood and adolescence–I. Age- and gender-specific prevalence. *Journal of Child Psychology and Psychiatry* 34:851-867.

D'Augelli, AR (1996), Lesbian, gay, and bisexual development during adolescence and young adulthood. In *Textbook of Homosexuality and Mental Health*. (Cabaj, R. & Stein, T., Eds.), Washington DC: American Psychiatric Press, Inc., pp. 267-288.

D'Augelli, AR & Hershberger SL (1993), Lesbian, gay, and bisexual youth in community settings: personal challenges and mental health problems. *Am J Community Psychol* 21:421-448.

Dawes, M, Dorn LD, Moss, HB, Yao, JK, Kirisci, L, Ammerman, RT, Tarter, RE (1999), Hormonal and behavioral homeostasis in boys at risk for substance abuse. *Drug and Alcohol Dependence*, 55:165-176.

DeBord, K,Wood, PK, Sher, KJ, Good, GE (1998), The relevance of sexual orientation to substance abuse and psychological distress among college students. *Journal of College Student Development*, 39(2):157-168.

Fulkerson, JA, Harrison, PA, Beebe, TJ (1999), DSM-IV substance abuse and dependence: are there really two dimensions of substance use disorders in adolescents?
Addiction, 94(4): 495-506.

Garofalo, R, Wolf, RC, Kessel, S, Palfrey, J, DuRant, RH (1998), The association
between health risk behaviors and sexual orientation among a school based sample of adolescents. *Pediatrics*, 101:895-902.

Graham, AW & Schultz, TK (1998), *Principles of Addiction Medicine, 2nd Ed*,
Chevy Chase, MD, American Society of Addiction Medicine, Inc.

Herdt, GM, & Boxer, AM (1993), *Children of Horizens: How Gay and Lesbian Teens
are Leading a New Way Out of the Closet*. Boston, MA: Beacon Press.

Johnston, LD (1998), Monitoring the Future Study (press release). Ann Arbor, MI,
University of Michigan.

Kaminer, Y (1994), *Adolescent Substance Abuse: A Comprehensive Guide to Theory
and Practice*. New York, NY: Plenum Press.

Kaminer, Y, & Burleson, J (1999), Psychotherapies for adolescent substance abusers:
15-month follow-up of a pilot study. *American Journal on Addictions*, 8(2)
114-119.

Lock, J & Steiner, H (1999), Gay, lesbian, and bisexual youth risks for emotional,
physical, and social problems: results from a community-based survey. *J. Am.
Acad. Child Adolescent Psychiatry*, 38(3) 297-304.

Myers, MG, Brown, SA, Vik, PW (1996), Adolescent substance use problems, In
Treatment of Childhood Disorders, 2nd, (EJ Mash & RA Barkley, Eds.) New
York, NY: Guilford Press, pp. 692-729.

Reinhertz, HZ, Giaconia, RM, Lefkowitz, ES, Pakiz, B, Frost, AK (1993), Prevalence of psychiatric disorders in a community population of older adolescents. *J.
Am. Acad. Child Adolescent Psychiatry*, 32:369-377.

Remafedi, G (1987), Adolescent homosexuality: psychosocial and medical implications. *Pediatrics*, 79(3) 331-337.

Remafedi, G, Farrow, JA, Deisher, RW (1991), Risk factors for attempted suicide in
gay and bisexual youth. *Pediatrics*, 87(6) 869-875.

Substance Abuse and Mental Health Services Administration (SAMHSA, 1993),
Screening and assessment of alcohol- and other drug-abusing adolescents: treat-
ment improvement protocol (TIP) series. U.S. Department of Health and Human
Services (93-2009).

Substance Abuse and Mental Health Services Administration (SAMHSA, 1995),
Guidelines for the treatment of Alcohol- and other drug-abusing adolescents:
treatment improvement protocol (TIP) series. U.S. Department of Health and
Human Services (95-3059).

APPENDIX 1

**Home Contract
Between Mom and Son**

Behavioral Guidelines	Closed/Open (negotiable)	Natural Consequences	Logical Consequences
No use of drugs/alcohol	Closed	Jail, IOP	In home arrest/no car until next clean screen
Curfew– 10pm weeknights 12:30pm weekends	Open	Lose sleep Mom worries	Curfew 2 hours earlier the next weekend and/or weekday
Keep grades above 2.0	Closed	No golf Limited college options	Lose weekend privileges, no sleepovers
Clean room 1 × per week	Open	Can't find things Clothes a mess Food leftovers– attract bugs	Won't be able to go out on Saturday until room is clean
Attend church or AA meeting once a week	Open	Spiritual side suffers – no support group	Attend both the next weekend to make up

Signatures:

Date: _____   Son _____   Mom_____

APPENDIX 2

Home Contract
Between Parents and Son

Behavioral Guidelines	Closed/Open (negotiable)	Natural Consequences	Logical Consequences
Clean tests	Closed	+ stay on track for goals – lose focus, lose money	+ more trust and responsibility – threat of intensive rehab (live-in)
Fulfilling legal obligations immediately MP class–2hr. class at Spectrum	Closed	+ save time and money – go to jail, lose money	+ more trust and responsibility – imposed by court
Maintaining Cs and above in every class When? (end of semester)	Closed	+ graduate from high school, happy with grades – don't graduate, fall behind	+ help with new car ($) help with spring trip – no help ($) for these things
Attention to surroundings (being polite, cleaning up, honest, performing community service) – lunch money – laundry	Open	+ help others, earn trust – don't gain privileges or trust	+ smoother relationships with family and community – increasing tension and unpleasantness at home
No work during the week	Closed	– I only make enough to last me a week, not to save	– Continued allowance for lunch $20.00

Signatures:

Date: _____   Son _____   Parent _____

The Importance
of Specialized Treatment Programs
for Lesbian and Gay Patients

Daniel Hicks, MD

SUMMARY. This article describes a dual diagnosis treatment program for the lesbian, gay, bisexual, and transgendered community in Washington, DC called the Lambda Center. By using a case example, the article describes how a specialized treatment program can more effectively treat and return a gay or lesbian patient to full functioning, by addressing specific issues which would be overlooked in a mainstream program. These unique issues include coming out, internalized homophobia, socialization, dating and intimacy for sexual minorities, use of certain recreational drugs, and the role of spirituality. The article also gives examples of failures and difficulties faced by lesbian and gay patients in straight programs. The author calls for further studies to prove the superior efficacy of specialized programs for lesbians and gay men and urges patients and providers demand that third party payers and HMOs authorize gay affirmative treatment programs because they are better for patients and probably more cost effective. *[Article copies available for a fee from The Haworth Document Delivery Service: 1-800-342-9678. E-mail address: <getinfo@haworthpressinc.com> Website: <http://www.HaworthPress.com>]*

KEYWORDS. Homosexuality, specialized treatment programs, gay and lesbian treatment, substance abuse treatment, recreational drug use, lesbian and gay mental health, internalized homophobia

Specialized addiction treatment programs provide a safe place for lesbian and gay persons to talk about all aspects of their lives without fear of criticism or judgement (Skinner and Otis 1992). This is a great relief for many

Dr. Daniel Hicks is affiliated with the Georgetown University Medical Center, Department of Psychiatry, 3780 Resevoir Road, Washington, DC 20007.

[Haworth co-indexing entry note]: "The Importance of Specialized Treatment Programs for Lesbian and Gay Patients." Hicks, Daniel. Co-published simultaneously in *Journal of Gay & Lesbian Psychotherapy* (The Haworth Medical Press, an imprint of The Haworth Press, Inc.) Vol. 3, No. 3/4, 2000, pp. 81-94; and: *Addictions in the Gay and Lesbian Community* (ed: Jeffrey R. Guss, and Jack Drescher) The Haworth Medical Press, an imprint of The Haworth Press, Inc., 2000, pp. 81-94. Single or multiple copies of this article are available from The Haworth Document Delivery Service [1-800-342-9678, 9:00 a.m. - 5:00 p.m. (EST). E-mail address: getinfo@haworthpressinc.com].

© 2000 by The Haworth Press, Inc. All rights reserved.

gay people in addiction treatment who have tended to segregate their lives, being in the closet at work or with their families, and only being out of the closet when they are at home or with friends. This can be a liberating experience for persons who are still struggling with acceptance of their identity and have few supports to openly discuss their feelings. It is also important that gay men and women find supportive and affirming groups outside of formal addiction treatment settings, such as lesbian and gay 12 step meetings or openly supportive meetings where it is safe to discuss their gay and lesbian issues without fear.

Specialized addiction treatment programs have experience dealing with the specific ways that substances are used in the gay and lesbian community, and which substances are somewhat unique to this community, which may not be understood in many mainstream programs. Specialized programs for gay men and lesbians can help people find alternative ways to socialize and be intimate without drugs or alcohol. They can also focus on safer sex education and responsible behavior, because HIV is so prevalent in the community and inextricably tied to substance use as risk factors. These programs also understand the coming out process, and how the conflicts in coming out often lead to substance abuse. This allows them to help the patient recognize internalized homophobia and find greater balance and self-acceptance. These programs also understand the role of spirituality for gays and lesbians in recovery, sometimes counteracting past damage caused by organized religion and offering an opportunity to open a spiritual path as part of the recovery process.

Because of oppression in society, lesbian and gay people are more prone to turn to substances for a variety of reasons. It is the goal of specialized treatment programs to understand these risks, and to be able to help patients not only become sober, but also to move on to greater self-acceptance and maturity. This involves overcoming self-preoccupation and fear caused by internalized homophobia, and shifting the focus to outside goals such as professional and career achievements, family and community, as well as increased political and church involvement.

In the last several years, more and more specialized programs offering mental health treatment for lesbian and gay people have emerged, especially those with substance abuse problems. It was recognized that relapse and failure seemed more common for many in the sexual minority community, because they were unable to express themselves openly and integrate the principles of recovery into their lives following treatment in mainstream programs. In many cases, lesbians and gay men were reluctant to enter into treatment because of fear of homophobia and prejudice. This paper will use a case example to demonstrate the effectiveness of a specialized treatment called the Lambda Center, and point out the unique interventions and knowledge which make these programs possibly more effective in reaching the gay or lesbian patient.

Michael was a 35-year-old professional gay white man who had recently begun to show signs of social withdrawal, irritability and erratic behavior. Lateness at work, missed appointments, and errors marred his usually excellent work performance. When friends tried to talk with him about these personality changes, he would become defensive and withdrawn. Finally, a group of close personal and professional friends gathered together to confront Michael about their concerns and encourage him to seek help. He finally admitted that his recreational cocaine and crystal methamphetamine use had begun spreading from the weekends into the weekdays, and was beginning to threaten his career. He accepted his friends' advice and agreed to seek treatment.

Michael had excellent insurance, and could go anywhere for treatment, but he chose a gay affirmative treatment program recommended by his friends. This was crucial to his recovery for several reasons. Many insurance companies would only authorize outpatient treatment for stimulant abuse, feeling that these drugs do not cause serious medical withdrawal, as is seen with alcohol or sedative detoxification, and therefore patients with addiction to stimulants could be safely treated in an outpatient program. These are common drugs of abuse in the gay community, and it is clear that they are intensely addictive. Because of this, the user often must be hospitalized for at least a few days, to break the cycle of use, and also allow the substance to begin clearing from their body. Specialized programs such as the Lambda Center are familiar with drugs endemic to the gay community. The Lambda Center has developed special relationships with third party payers that allow it to successfully obtain reimbursement for this more intensive treatment.

During these few days of treatment, dysphoria, restlessness, anxiety, and drug cravings emerged. It became clear that Michael was not only suffering from methamphetamine withdrawal, but also from Major Depressive Disorder, which is often hard to diagnose in the early stages of substance withdrawal. Michael had been in a seven-year relationship during which he occasionally used drugs and alcohol socially but never excessively. His lover had become involved with someone else and left about a year prior to admission. After the breakup, he coped with his depression by increasing his hours of work and isolating himself from many of his friends. This allowed him to move up rapidly in his firm due to his dedication and hard work. In order to relieve stress when he was not working and to cope with his loneliness, he had begun to go out every weekend and party excessively with drugs, dancing, and sex. He regularly traveled to "circuit parties" at various cities around the country. These consisted of long weekends of dancing and sex, fueled by recreational drugs such as ecstasy, Ketamine, cocaine, and crystal methamphetamine. His life consisted of work, going to the gym so he could look good at the parties, and intense dancing and drugs every weekend. There was little room for rest and relaxation, an intolerance for intense affect and an impaired ability for emotional intimacy.

Over time, his excessive weekend recreation began to make him more tired and less effective at work, so he started using a little cocaine and amphetamine to increase his energy and performance. This was only a temporary solution, and gradually the drug use increased. He began showing up late and becoming delinquent in meeting deadlines. This led his friends to confront this need for addiction treatment. As he withdrew from the drugs, his sadness, grief and depression over the loss of his relationship became more apparent. He was started on antidepressant medication for treatment of depressive symptoms and to help decrease drug cravings. In many mainstream programs, this depression may have been attributed only to withdrawal and never medicated, because the patient would not have been as open to discussing the losses in his life or their emotional significance.

HISTORY OF SPECIALIZED TREATMENT PROGRAMS FOR THE LGBT COMMUNITY

Specific treatment programs for gays and lesbians did not exist until 1986 with the formation of the PRIDE Institute (Ratner 1988). Although precise demographics about the lesbian and gay community are difficult to clearly delineate due to the fact that many persons are unwilling to self-identify, most studies do support the idea that there is an increased incidence of substance abuse in the lesbian and gay community (Erwin 1993). Estimates of incidence of addiction in this population range between 28-35%, compared with 10-12% in the heterosexual community (Cabaj 1996). One derogatory explanation is that homosexuality and alcoholism arose through a common pathological psychosexual developmental arrest; fortunately, this theory has been put to rest (Nardi 1982). As studies have inquired into the origins of homosexuality, it has been hypothesized that a gene for alcoholism, which clearly has a strong genetic component, may be in close proximity to a gene for homosexuality, so that a person who is homosexual may also be at higher risk to be alcoholic (Cabaj 1996).

More psychological explanations for the increased incidence of addiction in the gay and lesbian community describe addiction as a learned behavior, possibly superimposed upon a genetic predisposition (Ghindia and Kola 1996). For years, the only place to meet other lesbian or gay people safely (or at all) was in bars. This phenomenon still exists for many people today, especially in small towns where there are no gay neighborhoods or other social venues (Kelly 1994). If one spends enough time in an environment that encourages drinking and drug use, some individuals will develop a substance abuse problem, especially those with a genetic predisposition. For others with social anxieties or discomfort about having sex, drugs and alcohol may be experienced as necessary in order to relax enough to approach strangers, to socialize, or to perform sexually.

Another important factor in understanding addiction in the gay and lesbian community is both internalized and societal homophobia (Fleisher and Fillman 1995). Societal homophobia is also called heterosexism (Amico 1997). Homophobia is characterized by self-blame, a negative self-concept, and self directed anger. It is associated at times with self-destructive behaviors such as substance abuse, the development of a sense of victimization, feelings of inadequacy, hopelessness, and despair (Niesen and Sandall 1990). This inner self-hatred due to one's sexual feelings can interfere with psychological development, with drugs and/or alcohol providing escape from these negative feelings (Niesen, 1993). The phenomenon of increased substance abuse is often seen in oppressed communities, especially racial minorities and other socioeconomically oppressed groups.

STRUCTURE OF SPECIALIZED PROGRAMS

The program at the Lambda Center is a unique partnership between the Psychiatric Institute of Washington (DC) and the Whitman Walker Clinic, one of the nation's largest gay and lesbian health clinics. The Whitman Walker Clinic has become the District of Columbia's largest HIV service provider. The Lambda Center provides inpatient and partial hospitalization for the lesbian, gay, bisexual, and transgender community with psychiatric and/or substance abuse problems. The unit is on a locked ward with 8-10 beds, which also houses the partial hospitalization program for outpatients daily (Monday-Friday) from 10:00 AM to 3:30 PM. The program currently includes a psychoeducational group (Niesen 1997) which focuses on such topics as anger management, stress reduction, depression, medication, grief, safer sex, and HIV. A social worker, pastoral counselor, or nurse clinician leads this group. There is an expressive therapy group, led by an art therapist, in which patients work in a variety of expressive media: art, writing, storytelling, music therapy and sociodrama-type role playing. These therapeutic modalities seek to access emotions not always available through verbal or language based therapy. There is a break for lunch, then traditional process group psychotherapy, which works with current or past issues in a group format. Each day there is an addictions group, led by a Certified Addictions Counselor. These groups deal with such topics as: relapse triggers, relapse prevention, 12 step Meeting participation, relaxation/meditation techniques, the importance of social support for recovery, spirituality, and other issues related to recovery. The psychiatrist sees patients for psychiatric evaluation and treatment. Case management services are offered which provide assistance with social services, housing, and communication with families and work. Individual, family, and couples therapy may be done when indicated and time allows, but often this is coordinated with outside therapists. There is usually a morning and evening checkout time to support abstinence in the community and to provide planning for the evening and next day's activities. Individuals in treatment are strongly encouraged to attend 12 step or recovery meetings in the evenings and on weekends. Outpatients are encouraged to explore both gay and "straight" meetings in the community to develop a compatible recovery support system.

The staff is multidisciplinary with a psychiatrist as medical director and a program director who is an ordained minister and pastoral counselor. Also on staff are nurses, psychiatric technicians, an art therapist, social worker, and addiction counselor. Some members of the staff are straight and some gay; all staff are asked to be open about their sexual orientation and relationship status with patients. This is because honesty and openness are felt to be important for optimal health and recovery, and should be modeled by the staff whenever possible.

The non-gay staff is gay-affirmative, and all staff participate in regular in-service education about lesbian and gay issues, such as dating, safer sex and intimacy, gay male couples and lesbian couples, treatment of HIV disease, grief and loss, discrimination in the community, political advocacy, gay families and parenting, and other issues that emerge in the course of treatment. There are also plans to offer evening and weekend components of the treatment program in order to provide greater continuity and safety for inpatients and outpatients. These treatment times are important also for potential patients who work during the day, but need an Intensive Outpatient Program.

As demonstrated in the case example, patients may begin their treatment as inpatients for detoxification, safety and establishment of abstinence. They then move to the partial hospitalization program, living at home and coming to the Center for groups each day. If their living environment is unsafe due to strong relapse potential, they are encouraged to go into recovery housing, either through Whitman Walker Clinic or in the community. This increases the chances of successful recovery. Those who cannot access safe housing or who relapse repeatedly despite maximal treatment efforts are often referred to more restrictive long-term treatment programs in the community where patients are closely monitored and supervised for several months until their recovery is more stable.

Offering a continuum of treatment intensity ranging from inpatient to partial hospitalization also gives a much greater opportunity for monitoring of early abstinence and psychotropic medication effectiveness. Once patients' mood and recovery are more stable, their treatment session frequency is decreased, allowing them to return to work or other community activities.

Alternatively, the patient is referred to the intensive outpatient program, and may be seen on 2-5 days/week. This frequency is often helpful for further stabilization, and helps the patient remain focused on his or her recovery goals. In addition to options for housing for addictions and for HIV, our affiliation with Whitman Walker Clinic also gives access to a two day/week intensive evening addiction program that lasts for several months. Once the patient is functioning adequately, and in stable recovery, they may be referred for further treatment in their community, often including individual therapy and 12 step meetings. As in the case with Michael, the community program lasted several months, allowing him to have support as he came out at work and to his family.

Whitman Walker Clinic and Lambda Center also have access to a community-wide network of mental health providers who are willing to see patients for individual, couples, family, or group therapy. These gay affirmative practitioners are in private practice settings, and offer a broad spectrum of treatment expertise. Some offer a sliding scale fee. The Lambda Center offers monthly educational programs for providers in the community on various mental health topics including substance abuse, transgender issues, employment discrimination, domestic violence, gay and lesbian youth, trauma survivors, couples and family therapy, psychopharmacology and other issues pertinent to the community.

TREATMENT OPTIONS

Individuals are often limited in their choice of addiction treatment settings by their HMO or insurance company. Such restrictions may also limit the effectiveness of treatment if the program does not address the patient's specific needs (Garnets et al. 1997). One patient at the Lambda Center sought addiction treatment at several programs in his small town in Alabama. He had found them interesting and helpful, but he found himself listening to others and never really sharing his own life story: coming out after being married with children, and his difficulties in meeting and socializing without using alcohol. In a gay affirmative program, he was able to open up and talk about his life, and for the first time felt like he had really begun to recover. Another patient, who had been diagnosed with AIDS and was forced to retire soon after his initial HIV test, developed cocaine addiction to cope with his depression, illness, and drastic change in lifestyle. He entered the same treatment program on two occasions; he was very open about his sexuality and health status and even had his family involved in treatment. However, the patient continued to relapse and went from powder to crack cocaine, because the full weight of his depression in the face of AIDS was not recognized and treated in this mainstream treatment program. When he entered a specialized program, he was able to grieve the loss of his lover, his job, and his past professional achievements. He was able to work through family issues and become closer to his supportive family. He also began to explore his spirituality and worked toward finding a new level of satisfaction in life without drugs or a highly-paid career.

Some treatment programs, and some 12-step meetings have actually encouraged people not to talk about their homosexuality (Lewis and Jordan 1989) or their HIV disease. There was concern that it might cause too much disturbance to the other people in the group, or that it was not relevant to their addiction treatment (Green and Faltz 1991). Other programs may claim to be sensitive to gay and lesbian issues, but may not really understand the coming out process and the special issues faced by lesbian and gay people. Some openly gay people go to treatment programs and have no trouble being fully out of the closet and even may present as free of internalized homophobia. They may say to their therapists, "You don't understand what it's like in the gay community; everyone drinks," or "everyone gets high" or "you have to do this to fit in." The therapists and the treatment program need to identify and confront this common presentation of denial and avoidance of therapeutic interventions.

One clinician, a well-known specialist in addictions treatment, became very upset when it was suggested that two of his patients who were referred for a mainstream chemical dependency program for cocaine addiction, might be better served in a gay and lesbian dual diagnosis program. Both of the patients were openly gay men with HIV Disease who had much more in common with the other patients in the lesbian and gay program. This clinician insisted that "addiction is addiction" and that he had treated many lesbian and gay people as well as HIV positive persons in his addiction program and they had done well. There continues to be a common misperception by many clinicians and psychiatrists that all addiction treatment is equal, so that any standard treatment program should be equally effective, without looking at complicating co-morbid factors (Ubell and Sumberg 1992).

To gain access to gay and lesbian affirmative treatment, it is necessary for patients and clinicians to speak up to the insurance companies. Patients are encouraged to ask their HMOs and insurance companies for access to specialized programs and gay affirmative therapists. Many patients who have been in other treatment settings realize the importance of being able to integrate all aspects of their life in their treatment. The law of supply and demand will eventually encourage insurance companies to recognize the importance of gay and lesbian treatment for both inpatient and outpatient therapy, and so they will hopefully include gay specific programs and gay-identified therapists in their panels.

COMING OUT AND HOMOPHOBIA

Michael seemed to be fairly open and "out." He had had a long-term committed relationship, and most of his socialization was within the gay community. However, he had never integrated his personal, emotional life with his family of origin, nor had he really "come out" at work except to a few close, trusted friends. This compartmentalization of his life set up a state of tension and secrecy. He could not really talk about his personal life or relationship at work, and lived in some fear of what would happen if he were found out. He also avoided many interactions with his family except for periodic dutiful holiday visits home, which he enjoyed. He was warmly received by his family and friends, but never included his lover in his visits. When at home, he did not reveal much about his personal life in the city. These secrets led to a constant underlying state of anxiety, which eventually resulted in depression and turning to substances for relief.

As Michael's mood lifted in treatment and he felt better about himself, he began to realize the cost of keeping his life so segregated. He began to explore the idea of "coming out" more, both at work and with his family. Over time, he began to self-identify as gay at work where he was accepted and supported. His visibility and his efforts led his company to offer domestic partner benefits for gay and lesbian employees. He was also allowed to do pro bono work for his firm in the lesbian and gay community. With this success, he also came out to his family, first to a trusted sister, then to other siblings and then to his parents. With the help of his therapist and the work he had done in the groups, he was prepared for the emotional reactions of his family. He was able to provide them information and materials to help them understand homosexuality, and to answer their questions about his health and counter some of their religious arguments. He also told them about PFLAG (Parents, Friends and Families of Lesbians and Gays), and they became involved with their local chapter for further understanding. His visits home became easier, and his communication with them was much more open and fulfilling.

The process of coming out and coming to self-acceptance is a unique journey for lesbian and gay people. Society tends to negate and condemn persons with different sexual orientation, and these negative feelings become integrated into the psyches of lesbian and gay people. Recognizing and coming to terms with these sexual/emotional feelings creates a cognitive dissonance, and usually leads to some pain and distress. Some gay men and lesbians are able to confront and accept these feelings and move to acceptance without professional help; others become extremely depressed, even suicidal, or turn to drugs and alcohol for relief.

Coming out is a non-linear, often lifetime process of coming to full acceptance of one's sexuality. Some gay men such as Michael, feel they are "out," and seem to live a fairly open life, but still avoid certain painful or sensitive areas. That is why many lesbian and gay people move to gay ghettoes, where they can experience affirmation from other gay people, and avoid censure by family or close friends during the coming out process.

Adolescents struggling with their sexuality are at increased risk of suicide, or they turn to drugs and alcohol to escape (Schneider and Farberow 1989). Many lesbian and gay people become overly dependent on drugs and alcohol to ease their anxiety in the coming out process, to aid in socializing and early sexual experimentation (Kus 1988). They sometimes become dependent on alcohol or drugs to function sexually and socially. For others, like Michael, they may turn to drugs or alcohol to fit in with their social circle, or when they encounter losses and disappointments later in life. A mainstream program may not have been as able to help Michael recognize that his coming out process had been halted, similar to an early developmental arrest due to some life trauma. For him to continue to grow and develop, it was essential to be able to help him continue his coming out process and so achieve a greater degree of self-realization and self-acceptance.

SOCIAL ISSUES IN RECOVERY

For years, the main social and gathering place for lesbians and gay men have been bars–even when they were not safe and subject to police harassment. In many small towns and communities, bars continue to be the main social outlet for the lesbian and gay community. Since the development of alcohol dependence is thought to have a strong genetic component, and many gay and lesbian people still tend to associate in bars, a certain percentage of these people will develop substance abuse problems. Many lesbians and gay men have marked anxiety about their sexual interest and behavior, and alcohol becomes a way to lessen that anxiety and help people perform sexually; for some this leads to abuse or dependence. Others have a great deal of social anxiety and fear, having never learned how to "date." Once again, alcohol or drugs become a social lubricant, lowering anxiety and inhibitions. For some, this becomes the only means of socializing comfortably (McKirnan and Peterson 1989).

Another major issue in the gay male community is the marked emphasis on sexuality and physicality. One can see pictures of perfect bodies advertising bars, phone lines, bathhouses, classified ads, etc. This gives the impression that the majority of gay men are predominantly interested in the sexual aspects of being gay and the key to self-acceptance and contentment is to be highly physically attractive. Most gay men and lesbians are capable of having wonderful relationships and sex without dwelling excessively on physical beauty, which tends to evaporate with time. The focus on physicality is exemplified by the circuit party–a series of weekend gatherings in various cities throughout the year, which draw thousands of mostly affluent gay men who dance and have sex all weekend under the influence of a variety of alcohol and drugs. These began as a way to raise money for AIDS organizations, but developed into a tribal ritual. They are justified as a legitimate fund-raising venue, and as a well-earned outlet and reward for a community which has survived a plague. But this environment provides a new avenue for drugs into the community. These parties are settings which support the heavy use of drugs of abuse that are somewhat unique to the gay community: ecstasy, Ketamine, GHB, crystal methamphetamine and "poppers," as well as the ubiquitous alcohol, marijuana and cocaine. The emphasis on perfect bodies and the use of steroids first for wasting, decreased libido, and depression in HIV disease, and then for cosmetic reasons can generate increased sexual acting out, frequently with lowered regard for safety due to the influence of drugs. Because of the attractiveness and visibility of this segment of the gay male community, many others are undoubtedly being influenced to use "party" drugs and practice unsafe behavior, leading to further HIV transmission as well as substance abuse. This certainly drew in Michael, who began using to escape his work tensions and loneliness, to find relief and sexual gratification, but who became dependent on the drugs due to his depression and his underlying predisposition.

Another important risk factor for substance abuse among gays and lesbians is the shame and guilt around sexual behavior. Many people grow up with inhibitions about sex due to religious backgrounds or social upbringing. This is compounded further for lesbians and gay men who lack affirmations for their sexuality. Alcohol or drugs become a way to desensitize a person to the anxiety surrounding sexuality. For a percentage of people, this becomes the only way to be sexually active, and thus sets up the pattern of substance abuse or addiction.

SPIRITUALITY AND HOMOSEXUALITY

AA is still considered one of the most successful methods for overcoming alcoholism; other 12 step groups use similar approaches to address other addictions. AA began as a religious approach to recovery (Kominars 1987). Most 12-step programs are essentially spiritual paths. For many people in the lesbian and gay community, organized religion tends to be a difficult area, because mainstream religions have tended to reject and condemn homosexuality. For many gay and lesbian people, this rejection creates an insurmountable problem, so they are reluctant to pursue 12 step programs that appear religious in nature. It is essential that treatment programs recognize that some lesbian and gay people come from very religious or spiritual backgrounds, but after coming out, found that their church rejected them. Due to this cognitive dissonance between their church and their sexuality, these gay people choose to walk away from organized religion, and often harbor bitterness. This is reinforced by the fact that fundamentalist religions continue to be the strongest spokespersons against gay people.

Many lesbian and gay people are very spiritual, despite the damage done to them by the church. There are many gay clergy, and many churches are openly embracing lesbian and gay people in their congregations and their leadership, especially in choir and music. But many people with substance abuse problems are estranged from their religion and oppose any discussion of spirituality. They often resist attending 12 step meetings because there is talk about "God," and some meetings are experienced as judgmental and condemning of gays and lesbians. Specialized treatment programs are aware of these conflicts, but also know the importance of spiritual repair in recovery. To address this, the program needs to help patients expand their concept of God, religion, faith, and spirituality. It is valuable in recovery to support the process of being open to exploring various religions, and entering one's own journey to find a power or force greater than one's self. This is the basis of spirituality; some people can find these answers in organized religion, but others need to find their own spiritual path.

CONCLUSION

Specialized treatment programs for lesbians and gay men are a relatively recent phenomenon. Although there are not enough controlled studies to demonstrate effectiveness, it is clear to many who work in these programs that they seem to be more powerful in helping patients achieve recovery and healing. Specialized treatment programs provide a safe space for sexual minority persons with substance abuse and emotional problems to talk about their lives freely. The issues discussed may have little or nothing to do with their sexual orientation, but the groups provide a sense of acceptance and support. The issues discussed may have little or nothing to do with their sexual orientation, but the groups provide a sense of acceptance and support, which may be a new experience for these patients. This nurturing environment allows patients to share secrets and pain they have often kept hidden. In being able to look at these issues, many personas can face painful issues and reach some resolution and healing so that they become stronger and more likely to stay sober when faced with new problems.

The strength of the specialized programs seems to be in providing a safe space for gay men and lesbians to confront problems in a community of support. A gay-affirming and supportive treatment program can help people resolve past issues such as incest and abuse, as well as foster the coming out process and self-acceptance. These programs offer the opportunity to address socialization skills, dating and intimacy issues, as well as HIV, grief and loss.

Specialized programs are sensitive to the damage experienced by many gays and lesbians within organized religion, and aid patients in finding their spiritual center.

Because of the special issues that the lesbian and gay community faces, it is important to fight for specialized programs and affirmative treatments. Hospitals, insurance carriers and third party payers should be requested to provide access to these programs. Further research needs to be done to prove their effectiveness, so that payers will realize they should be funded.

REFERENCES

Amico, J.M., & Niesen, J. (1997), Sharing the secret: the need for gay-specific treatment, *The Counselor*, May/June.

Cabaj, R.P. (1996), Substance abuse in gay men, lesbians, and bisexuals, *Textbook of Homosexuality and Mental Health*, Cabaj and Stein, Eds., Chap. 47, 783-800, APPI Press.

Erwin, K. (1993), Interpreting the evidence: competing paradigms and the emergence of lesbian and gay suicide as a social fact, *International Journal of Health Services*, 23(3): 437-453.

Fleisher, J., & Fillman, J. (1995), Lesbian and gay youth: treatment issues, *The Counselor*, Jan-Feb, 27-28.

Garnets, L., & Hancock, K.A. (1991), Issues in psychotherapy with lesbians and gay men: a survey of psychologists, *American Psychologist*, 46(9): 964-972.

Ghindia, D.J., & Kola, L.A. (1996), Co-factors affecting substance abuse among homosexual men, *Drug and Alcohol Dependence*, 41(3): 167-177.

Green, D., & Faltz, B. (1991), Chemical dependency and relapse in gay men with HIV infection, *Counseling Chemically Dependent People with HIV Illness*, The Haworth Press, Inc., 79-90.

Kelly, J. (1994), Preventing alcohol and other drug problems in the lesbian and gay community, California Department of Alcohol and Drug Programs, Sacramento, March.

Kominars, S.B. (1989), *Accepting ourselves: the 12 step journey of recovery for gay men and lesbians*, New York: Harper and Row.

Kus, R.J. (1988), Alcoholism and non-acceptance of gay self: the critical link, *Journal of Homosexuality*, 15(1-2): 25-41.

Kus, R.J. (1992), Spirituality in everyday life: experiences of gay men of alcoholics anonymous, *Journal of Chemical Dependency Treatment*, 5(1): 49-66.

Lewis, G.R., & Jordan, S.M. (1989), Treatment of the gay or lesbian alcoholic, *Alcoholism and Substance Abuse in Special Populations*, Lawson and Lawson, Eds., Aspen Publishers, Rockville, MD.

McKirnan, D.J., & Peterson, P.L. (1989), Psychosocial and cultural issues in alcohol and drug abuse: an analysis of a homosexual community, *Addiction Behaviors*, 14(5): 555-563.

Nardi, P. (1982), Alcoholism and homosexuality: a theoretical perspective, *Journal of Homosexuality*, 7(1): 9-25.

Niesen, J., & Sandall, H. (1990), Alcohol and other drug abuse in a gay/lesbian population: related to victimization? *Journal of Psychology & Human Sexuality*, 3(1): 151-168.

Niesen, J. (1993), Healing from cultural victimization: recovery from shame due to heterosexism, *Journal of Gay & Lesbian Psychotherapy*, 2(1): 49-63.

Niesen, J. (1997), An inpatient psychoeducational model for gay men and lesbians with alcohol and drug abuse problems, *Chemical Dependency Treatment: Innovative Group Approaches*, L.D. McVinney, Binghamton, The Haworth Press, Inc. 37-51.

Ratner, E. (1988), Model for the treatment of lesbian and gay alcohol abusers, *Alcoholism Treatment Quarterly*, 5(1/2): 25-46.

Schneider, S.G., & Farberow, N.L. et al., (1989), Suicidal behavior in adolescent and young adult gay men, *Suicide and Life-Threatening Behavior*, 19(4): 381-94.

Skinner, W., & Skinner, O. (1992), Drug use among lesbian and gay people: findings, research, design, insights, and policy issues from the trilogy project, *The Research Symposium on Alcohol and Other Drug Problem Prevention Among Lesbians and Gay Men: Proceedings*, October.

Ubell, V., & Sumberg D. (1992), Heterosexual therapists treating homosexual addicted clients, *Journal of Chemical Dependency Treatment*, 5(1):19-33.

A Memoir of Homosexuality, Psychiatry, Chemical Dependence, Depression and Recovery: Confessions of a Social Activist

Anonymous

SUMMARY. In recounting his interactions with psychiatry–in psychotherapy, as an openly gay candidate for residency, with depression and in recovery from chemical dependence–the author, who is a gay and social activist, physician and writer, offers perspective on the impact of psychiatry on the trajectory of social change. *[Article copies available for a fee from The Haworth Document Delivery Service: 1-800-342-9678. E-mail address: <getinfo@haworthpressinc.com> Website: <http://www.HaworthPress.com>]*

KEYWORDS. Addiction, depression, Alcoholics Anonymous, physicans in recovery

When I was in residency training in anesthesiology in Boston in the mid-1970s, I saw my first psychotherapist, an overtly homophobic Harvard Medical School faculty psychiatrist. He had the following response to my

[Haworth co-indexing entry note]: "A Memoir of Homosexuality, Psychiatry, Chemical Dependence, Depression and Recovery: Confessions of a Social Activist." Anonymous. Co-published simultaneously in *Journal of Gay & Lesbian Psychotherapy* (The Haworth Medical Press, an imprint of The Haworth Press, Inc.) Vol. 3, No. 3/4, 2000, pp. 95-103; and: *Addictions in the Gay and Lesbian Community* (ed: Jeffrey R. Guss, and Jack Drescher) The Haworth Medical Press, an imprint of The Haworth Press, Inc., 2000, pp. 95-103. Single or multiple copies of this article are available from The Haworth Document Delivery Service [1-800-342-9678, 9:00 a.m. - 5:00 p.m. (EST). E-mail address: getinfo@haworthpressinc.com].

© 2000 by The Haworth Press, Inc. All rights reserved.

trying to have a sense of humor–a common defense mechanism among gay men and lesbians, Jews, Blacks and other minorities facing prejudice–about painful childhood memories of cross-dressing: "I've heard all fourteen homosexual jokes." During that same time, I was channel surfing one afternoon and chanced upon a local talk show that featured one of the first openly gay psychiatrists in America. The next day I switched psychiatrists. In terminating the earlier therapy, I confronted that psychiatrist with the issue of his prejudice in what was perhaps my first act as a gay and social activist. Without realizing it, I had crossed a threshold that would determine the trajectory of the rest of *my* life.

Had I known then the cost of giving such priority to my activism–to being able to tell the truth as best I knew and believed it and to fight for that right and for equality and respect, I might have hesitated. In any case, in explaining my decision to the Harvard psychiatrist, who was just returning from giving "expert" testimony in a court case, I predicted that in the future, psychiatrists such as himself who were overtly homophobic would become the subjects of malpractice litigation. I predicted the same fate for other clinicians involved with coercion therapies and other efforts at sexual orientation change. Twenty-five years later, notwithstanding statements deploring such therapies by the American Psychiatric Association, the American Psychological Association and even the American Psychoanalytic Association, there has been only a trickle of such cases. Nothing like a trend has yet been established. Meanwhile, the size of the market for sexual orientation change therapy within psychiatry remains unknown.

In the heyday of his influence as the leading figure of our era on the complex of issues and phenomena he himself refers to, albeit in quotes, as "sissyness," I confronted Richard Green. He is the author of a number of influential studies and books, the best known of which is *The "Sissy-Boy Syndrome" and the Development of Homosexuality* from Yale University Press. He was also a key figure in the declassification of homosexuality as a mental disorder in 1973-74. I asked him whether psychiatry had merely changed its strategy from diagnosing and treating "homosexuality" to diagnosing and treating "the gender identity disorder of childhood." He wouldn't hazard a guess. Though clearly an ally of the gay community in his championing the APA declassification (and in subsequent work on homosexuality, ethics and the law), he had otherwise kept his distance from the gay liberation movement. On the one occasion he finally and reluctantly agreed to be interviewed for the gay press (the conversation with me was conducted by telephone), he was clearly uncomfortable and guarded. One conclusion of his work on "sissy" boys is that some of them, with the right parenting, role models, and guidance, can escape that syndrome and graduate (my word) to normal (my word) sexual life. Were *you* one of the sissy boys you are studying? I finally asked Green bluntly. He wouldn't comment, of course. Whether or not he had been a "sissy" who managed to *achieve* heterosexual "normality" was understood by Green to be a personal question; similarly, questions regarding the impact of his study on the gay community were appreciated as political. They were not seen as integral to the studies nor as viewpoints that were presented as exclusively scientific. Not that Green wasn't/isn't right about at least *some* "sissy" boys. It's just that his reserve, his wanting to distance himself from the gay community as it was unfolding socially and politically, was intriguing and seemed in real contrast, for example, to the accessibility of Judd Marmor. A few years earlier, Marmor, a former President of the American Psychiatric Association who was a chief figure in the APA declassification of homosexuality, had edited a collection, *Homosexual Behavior: A Modern Reappraisal.* Even though Marmor could likewise reveal defensiveness through his abiding regard for the work of his colleague Irving Bieber (a major, homophobic critic of the APA declassification), he was open to dialogue in a way and to an extent that Green was not. Beyond his considerable work affirming civil liberties and ethics within a context of contemporary and regional social mores, Green, it is difficult not to conclude, ultimately rests his case for "the development of homosexuality"–in *some* boys and, by implication, in more than some–on syndromes of psychopathology.

In the late 1970s, I opted to do a second residency–in psychiatry– and to come out during interviews in various programs. This was several years following the removal of the category of "homosexuality" from DSM-III, yet the homophobia I encountered in some of America's leading departments of psychiatry, detailed in my very first essay for the gay press (entitled "Trial By Ordeal" for *Gay Community News*), was worse than anything I could have imagined. One interviewer put his feet up on the table about two inches from my face and began munching from a bag of nuts. After several minutes of this, he said to me: "Do you see what I'm doing here? I'm eating my own nuts right here in front of you. What do you think about that?" Another said to me, the sarcasm dribbling from his lips: "Tell me now, what does your mother think about you?" As earlier described, my initiation as a gay activist took place when I decided to leave my homophobic psychiatrist for one who was himself a gay activist. The catalyst for the next big step in my activism was this experience of interviewing for the residency in psychiatry. A lot of my best efforts and energies went into independent writing, most of it journalism, including a stint as the editor of a newsletter for the first group of openly gay and lesbian psychiatrists, as well as other organizational and political activities. Supporting myself with part-time work in outpatient addiction medicine (methadone maintenance), I became a watchdog for what was going on in psychiatry around the issue of homosexuality.

Most of my pieces were about how traditional psychiatric viewpoints, still being proffered by reactionary forces working to overturn the APA declassification, were being superceded in scientific and public discourse by those of sex research/sexology–e.g., the Masters and Johnson study, *Homosexuality in Perspective*. When it was published in 1979, it created a firestorm of controversy, with gay activists as well as with psychiatrists and the public at large. From my perspective, the most salient thing about it is that it usurped turf previously held by psychiatry. It was a pivotal example of the passage of authority from psychiatry to other disciplines on a subject that psychiatry, until then, had "owned." Psychiatry had in real measure in fact created the idea of "homosexuality" as a diagnosis and condition to be treated. In addition to a recounting of my experience of coming out during interviews for residency in psychiatry, reviewing *Homosexuality in Perspective* was in fact one of my first projects as a gay activist and journalist. It was my first book review. Accompanying it was my first interview for the gay press (with M&J, for *The Advocate*).

Eventually, I would discover an even larger trend engulfing sex research as well as psychiatry, at least with regard to homosexuality: the passage of authority from outsider/mostly heterosexual medical and scientific "experts" to the voices and studies of gay and lesbian scholars and writers ourselves. Would the same trend eventually reveal itself with regard to addiction and depression, two other realms that were to claim me as citizen? That is, would our understanding of addiction and depression eventually emerge more from the voices and experiences and actions of insiders–of those suffering from those afflictions–than from the professional "experts," mostly outsiders, studying them?

In those days, I had become what I myself called an "anti-psychiatrist," a Szaszian critic of what I called, during the period when I got to know and interview Thomas Szasz, "the Sovietization of American psychiatry." Eventually, my skepticism about psychiatry gave way to a broader-based skepticism about medicine and science in general. That is, I questioned the ability of "science," of scientific knowledge and methods, to change prejudice in individuals and society, and to effect social change. Very naively, I'd believed that, beyond the declassification of homosexuality as a mental disorder by the APA, if such popular and respected "scientists" as Masters and Johnson next reassured the world that homosexuality was not any kind of mental disorder, the world would quickly abandon its long-held prejudices. The firsthand experience of the failure of that to take place was a turning point for me. Gradually, I came to believe less-and-less devoutly in the sanctity and reliability of medicine and science. In fact, the more I looked into the history of those two enterprises, the more I realized that they were in league with and service to oppressive and irrational forces at least as often as they were not. I had come some distance from the faith in science as religion that I had held in medical school and later in residency training at what was considered the world's most prestigious hospital. My attitude towards art, incidentally, would follow a similar trajectory. Just as I had taken as gospel everything said or done in the names of science, I likewise tended to venerate anything sanctified as "art," a situation that was to change impressively with coming to grips with what I was to call my "adult knowledge" of composer Richard Wagner. Notwithstanding these caveats and my negative experiences, I had enough perspective and regard for the profession otherwise that I remained in and out of psychotherapy, consistently with psychiatrists.

Meanwhile, as my work as a gay- and, soon enough, AIDS-activist consumed more and more of my energies, my dependence on alcohol, marijuana and cigarettes likewise grew. In the spring of 1983, I was burnt out, as we say in common parlance, and hospitalized with a major depressive episode. The background of my psychiatrist is pertinent to this discussion. During the period when I was spiraling into this vortex of depression, I was in therapy with a gay-affirmative psychiatrist who had in fact worked with a number of gay activists of renown, including my life partner, whose mother had referred her son in the hope of having him "cured" of his homosexuality. Little did she (or for that matter the psychiatrist himself) know that he was a pioneer in helping gay men to see and believe that they and gay were good, that social activism was the right path. Unwittingly, in his work with his patients, he had stimulated that process of overt social activism that he, being from the previous generation, hadn't had the resources or timing or courage (in a far more harshly repressive era) to pursue himself. With neither self-awareness as such nor subsequently ever credited as such, he was likewise a pioneer of the work and perspectives of what was first called the Gay Caucus of Members of the American Psychiatric Association (a name the APA forced the fledgling group to change), and eventually as the Association of Gay and Lesbian Psychiatrists. In the mid-1980s, a fiercely activist play about gay men and AIDS was dedicated to him.

So this psychiatrist, an analyst, was a real *mensch* who was especially helpful to me in coming to grips not only with my calling as a writer and my mission as an activist but also with my Jewish identity, which I had eschewed to the point of pathology. On the other hand, he was older and out-of-touch with the management of clinical depression. Worse, but like most of his psychiatric colleagues, he knew next to nothing about alcoholism and chemical dependence. Nowadays we do have what are informally known as "addiction psychiatrists." Yet even today, in this era of harm reduction, most psychiatrists/psychotherapists want to have little to do with overt addicts and often shun training in addiction to the extent that they are amazingly unaware of earlier and subtler signs of addiction.

So there I was, spiraling into a major depression with a psychiatrist who'd done this wonderful work with gay activists but who was a Horneyan analyst untrained in treating clinical depression and knowing even less about chemical dependence. What were we going to do? Fortunately, I had enough presence of mind to diplomatically ask him to get another psychiatrist, one who was hospital-based, to consult on my case, and in fact to take over the management of my depression, which was going to require hospitalization. In this leading New York City Hospital, I was placed on imipramine, which took weeks to take effect. I came within moments of receiving ECT. None of the consulting psychiatrists on my case, including the chairman of the department, had any sense of the very central, pivotal role that chemical dependence was playing in my circumstances.

The Horneyan analyst had known of my use of alcohol and marijuana but had conspired with me, as did the others, to minimize it. For one thing, at the time of my hospitalization, I was so depressed that I had ceased using these substances months earlier. No one had any idea that years of chronic marijuana use can cause major depression, that depression and paranoia are major and common side effects of marijuana use. And everyone accepted that my "periodic" use of these substances meant that I wasn't a typical addict. They had no idea that "control" by quitting–periodicity–is a principal and classic pattern of addiction.

Following my hospitalization, I was on prescribed imipramine and Xanax for about six months, during which time I remained abstinent from alcohol and marijuana. At the time of my release, there was no advice regarding recovery or even abstinence. I resumed therapy with my analyst, who, sadly, was in the early stages of Alzheimer's Disease, which accelerated rapidly with the death of his life partner of 30 years. I then switched to the psychiatrist who had managed my depression in the hospital and with whom I remained in intermittent psychotherapy until his retirement some fifteen years later. We would do periods of short-term, goal-oriented therapy and I never required medication of any kind again.

The principal reason I didn't require medication subsequent to my hospitalization and initial treatment for depression is that, independent of my psychiatrists and my psychotherapy, I had, on my own, discovered the optimal treatment for my condition: recovery. This term refers in general to the recovery movement that encompasses programs based upon the 12-steps and related literatures originally conceived for Alcoholics Anonymous. Fortunately, over my years of medical training, my antennae had keyed into drug addiction and recovery. I had become aware that when it came to genuine abstinence and recovery, as opposed to harm reduction, there was only one treatment that had ever shown any real success: Alcoholics Anonymous. After nearly a year of self-imposed abstinence but not in a program of recovery, I relapsed and made a discovery of a pattern that was pathognomonic of my own alcoholism, a characteristic of this disease I had first learned about during my internship rotation through an alcohol detoxification ward: progression. In the thirteen months since my last drink, my ability to consume alcohol had somehow doubled. And there was another development, a symptom that enabled me to make the diagnosis of alcoholism on my patient, who happened to be me: I had my first blackout. Recognizing the symptoms on my own, and with virtually no insight or support from my psychiatrists during this period, I diagnosed myself as an alcoholic and drug addict and entered into recovery, where I have been sober for over fifteen years, a day at at time. (Later, I would discover that the problem of sexual compulsivity in my life likewise needed to be engaged via recovery.) In the early period of my recovery, when I confronted the psychiatrist who had managed my depression and with whom I remained in and out of therapy until his retirement last year, he responded with an honesty that cemented our therapeutic relationship. He apologized and said that, like most other psychiatrists, he had never learned much about addiction and chemical dependence, and knew even less about 12-step recovery. He hadn't known better, he said.

Eventually, I settled into the field of what we now call addiction medicine, and my viewpoints have not changed. Though we engage broadly and diversely in what we call harm-reduction, and continue to experiment with a variety of other approaches and medications, those in the field, including addiction psychiatrists, concur that the only approach with demonstrable success in achieving *abstinence* from chemical dependence continues to be 12-Step recovery. The nature of the program, with its core principles of spirituality and anonymity, is such that scientific studies establishing that success remain elusive.

For the self-identified gay man or lesbian in recovery who wishes to supplement his program with outpatient psychotherapy and/or treatment, the outlook is good, but there are pitfalls–e.g., from the sense of competition the psychotherapist may feel from the recovery program. In many instances, clients will be able to work through life issues and crises primarily by utilizing his tools of recovery, perhaps to the extent that the need for the therapy will be minimized or even eliminated.

The other area of concern here that could arise in psychotherapy for a gay client in recovery is homophobia in that world or environment. Despite individual experiences of homophobia and other prejudices at some meetings, such reports seem remarkably few and the integration of gay men and lesbians into the fabric of the recovery community is an impressive demonstration of the principles and power of this spiritual program based upon anonymity, and one of whose slogans is "principles before personalities." In most locales there are meetings, often many, specifically designated as gay and/or lesbian.

So how can this diverse experience come together in coherent perspective?

I propose that these three major areas of experience share a common ground, as they have interfaced with psychiatry–homosexuality, chemical dependence and depression–when they are placed in social, political and historical context. Just as psychiatry and psychotherapy did not and still do not have the sociopolitical answers to the problems of a homophobic society and world, they do not have the answers to another major realm of experience and problems that afflicts not only gay men, but all of humankind: addiction. Notwithstanding the smaller affirmative contributions of countless individual psychotherapists to the consciousness and self-affirmation of countless individuals, nowhere more than in the failure of psychiatry and psychotherapy in regard to homosexuality is it more clear that the solutions are neither medical nor psychiatric so much as social. These solutions are what people in recovery would designate as "spiritual," and political, in the sense that great changes in social thinking are needed to effect social change on a mass scale. This scale is perforce political, involving new priorities for funding, new legislation and the leadership to bring it about. In other words, the experience of psychiatry in these realms offers another proof of the old adage that the personal is political, and vice versa: What seems so personal, individual, medical and psychiatric turns out to be so underpinned socially and culturally that it is inevitably political.

Whatever the role of psychiatry in stimulating observation and ferment in intellectual discourse, whatever the role of individual psychotherapy in priming some social activists, the treatment for homophobia has turned out to be a social revolution called gay liberation, which is in turn entangled within greater sexual revolutions. In the same way, the treatment for "hysteria" ultimately turned out to be not a pill or a therapeutic approach but a social revolution called feminism. Likewise, the most successful treatment to date for addiction has turned out to be a social-spiritual movement called recovery. Will the same pattern eventually reveal itself with regard to the other principal realm of my experience with psychiatry–depression? My guess is that the answer will prove to be yes. The *greatest* breakthrough in treating depression won't turn out to be personal/individual (some new form of individual or group psychotherapy) or biochemical (some new anti-depressant or family thereof). Rather, it will be sociopolitical, a revolution of economic, cultural and social priorities and systems, some quantum leap of change in a future in which humankind's most fundamental needs are better understood, and met.

REFERENCES

Bieber, I., Dain, H., Dince, P., Drelich, M., Grand, H., Gundlach, R., Dremer, M., Rifkin, A., Wilbur, C., and Bieber, T. (1962), *Homosexuality: A Psychoanalytic Study*. New York: Basic Books.
Green, R. (1987), *The "Sissy Boy Syndrome" and the Development of Homosexuality*. New Haven, CT: Yale University Press.

Marmor, J., Ed. (1980), *Homosexual Behavior: A Modern Reappraisal*. New York: Basic Books.

Masters, W. H. and Johnson, V. E. (1979), *Homosexuality in Perspective*. New York: Little, Brown.

Szasz, T. (1965), Legal and moral aspects of homosexuality. In *Sexual Inversion: The Multiple Roots of Homosexuality*, ed. J. Marmor. New York, New York: Basic Books, pp 124-139.

Szasz, T. (1974), *The Myth of Mental Illness: Foundations of a Theory or Personal Conduct*, Revised Edition. New York: Harper & Row.

Sex Like You Can't Even Imagine: "Crystal," Crack and Gay Men

Jeffrey R. Guss, MD

SUMMARY. The past five years have witnessed a great increase in the use of the stimulant drugs crystal methamphetamine and smoked cocaine (crack) as part of a pattern of hypersexual behavior inextricably interwoven with substance dependence. With these patients, the problems are not independent, and exist almost exclusively in the company of one another. The paper describes a framework for evaluating patients and assessing their readiness for treatment in office based individual treatment that is informed by psychoanalytic principles. Typical resistances at each stage of treatment are described, with clinical recommendations for management. Common transference and countertransference paradigms are described. The paper includes psychoanalytic exploration of the possible meanings of the experience of drug/sex addiction, abstinence and fantasies that often precede relapse. *[Article copies available for a fee from The Haworth Document Delivery Service: 1-800-342-9678. E-mail address: <getinfo@haworthpress inc.com> Website: <http://www.HaworthPress.com>]*

KEYWORDS. Crystal methamphetamine, crack cocaine, sexual addiction homosexuality, psychoanalytic, transference

Dr. Jeffrey R. Guss is a Candidate, New York University Postdoctoral Program in Psychotherapy and Psychoanalysis; Clinical Assistant Professor of Psychiatry, New York University School of Medicine; and maintains a private practice in analytic psychotherapy as well as the treatment of addictive disorders.

The author wishes to thank the following for their invaluable contributions to the development of this article: Jack Drescher, MD, Robert Glick, MD, Steven Hartman, PhD, Nathan Kravis, MD, Virginia Kelley, PhD, and Eric Gabriel Lehman.

[Haworth co-indexing entry note]: "Sex Like You Can't Even Imagine: 'Crystal,' Crack and Gay Men." Guss, Jeffrey R. Co-published simultaneously in *Journal of Gay & Lesbian Psychotherapy* (The Haworth Medical Press, an imprint of The Haworth Press, Inc.) Vol. 3, No. 3/4, 2000, pp. 105-122; and: *Addictions in the Gay and Lesbian Community* (ed: Jeffrey R. Guss, and Jack Drescher) The Haworth Medical Press, an imprint of The Haworth Press, Inc., 2000, pp. 105-122. Single or multiple copies of this article are available from The Haworth Document Delivery Service [1-800-342-9678, 9:00 a.m. - 5:00 p.m. (EST). E-mail address: getinfo@haworthpressinc.com].

© 2000 by The Haworth Press, Inc. All rights reserved.

INTRODUCTION

What is the role of substance use in the expression of sexuality? What is the role of sexuality in drug use? In my practice, I work with many gay men as they go through the difficult process of the discovery or acknowledgement of their drug/alcohol addictions, exploration of the intimate relationship that drug and alcohol use has with their sexuality and identity, the decision to change this relationship and the process of recovery. When sex and drugs are powerfully linked, abstaining from drug use inevitably brings about an exploration of sexuality in sobriety, often nostalgically haunted by memories of drug-fuelled sex. Each phase of recovery from addiction (acceptance, establishment of abstinence, relapse prevention and recovery) brings up profound experiences evoking difficult, often confounding questions. Clinical aspects of treatment to be discussed include: the patient's motivations for abstinence, relapse triggers unique to this population, exploration of sexuality in the therapeutic process, and frequent transference paradigms. This paper will not address such categorical issues as the incidence or "reasons" for addiction in the gay community as a whole. Rather, it will present an office-based clinical model for treating a particular population: gay men for whom intense, compulsive stimulant drug use combined with sex has become a problem.

Addiction in this context is most often manifested by severe affective disruption following episodes of use, loss of control of drug intake, an excess of money and time spent pursuing sex and drugs, and the constriction of other kinds of meaningful engagement in life. This treatment approach is abstinence-based, uses conventional early recovery techniques, and is informed by psychoanalytic ideas and understanding, although not "traditional" analytic treatment techniques. This paper will not offer advice about the "best" treatment modalities for certain drug addictions because these categorical recommendations (inpatient rehabilitation, intensive outpatient programs for this or that drug addiction) may not be indicated, acceptable or available to certain patients. In addition to problems of patient preference or access, many patients come to outpatient treatment unprepared for the commitment to abstinence required for initiation of programmatic (group) treatment, intensely fearful of giving up their drug/sexual experiences. Becoming ready, then making this commitment becomes the initial focus of the therapy.

HOMOSEXUALITY, PSYCHOANALYSIS AND ADDICTION: STRANGE AND ESTRANGED BEDFELLOWS

There is a long and contentious history of psychoanalytic theory and practice in the understanding and treatment of both drug addiction and homosexuality. Both areas of clinical focus historically proved to be extravagantly unresponsive to traditional analytic approaches in terms of changing behavior explicitly defined as pathological. Because of the persistence of homosexual desire and active addiction in patients treated for these conditions while in treatment based in drive/conflict theory, analysts assigned a severe degree of psychopathology to each. This culminated in the declaration of their untreatability, with diagnosis of psychotic or severe sociopathic character pathology in both populations. At the same time, psychoanalytic approaches to addictions have long been seen as dangerous and "enabling" from the traditional addiction treatment community. John Wallace (1978) described the ways that insight and therapeutic "neutrality" supported the denial that enabled continued drinking and the inevitable progression of the addiction. He described psychotherapy itself as a betrayal of the patient, its use reflecting the clinician's lack of understanding of the principles of addiction treatment. There has, however, been a steady trickle of insightful writing on addictions by psychoanalysts. Such clinicians and writers as Edward Khantzian, Leon Wurmser, Henry Krystal and Lance Dodes have made valuable contributions to the field, and offer useful insights into working with addicted individuals in analytic settings. A concise review of their ideas can be found in Jon Morgenstern and Jeremy Leed's article, "Contemporary Psychoanalytic Theories of Substance Abuse: A Disorder in Search of a Paradigm" (Morgenstern and Leeds, 1993) and more recently, "Three Perspectives on Addiction," by Brian Johnson (1999). Some of these ideas will be introduced in the later part of this paper.

There is a long history of animosity from gay-affirmative psychotherapists toward the old guard of psychoanalysis, challenging and rejecting the psychoanalytic pathologizing of homosexuality. The misunderstanding and oppression of homosexuality by American psychoanalysis has been extensively described elsewhere (Lewes, 1988) and will not be recounted here. The readers are no doubt familiar with the slow and agonizing process by which homosexuality has been removed from our core text of psychiatric disorders, the Diagnostic and Statistical Manual. The American Psychoanalytic Association as well has changed its official position, if not the hearts and minds of all its members, regarding the designation of homosexuality per se as pathologic. Therefore, it is increasingly clear that it is not homosexuality per se that we explore analytically in work with these patients, but the function of the intense, obsessive drug/sex behavior in terms of object relations and self experience.

WHY DO GAY MEN LOVE COCAINE AND CRYSTAL METHAMPHETAMINE?

Stimulant drugs, particularly cocaine and methamphetamine ("crystal"), are particularly appealing to gay men in a highly sexualized subculture that exists within the broader gay community. The acute physical effects of meth-amphetamine include an increase in sensory acuity and energy and a decrease in appetite, as well as a lowered need for sleep. Acute psychological effects include an increase in confidence, verbosity, and alertness, grandiosity, self-idealization and euphoria. There is a marked elevation in mood and sex drive, as well as a decrease in boredom, loneliness and timidity (Ling, p. 13, 1998). Cocaine initially produces a sense of increased alertness and sense of well being. It lowers anxiety and social inhibitions and heightens energy, self-esteem and the positive emotions aroused by interpersonal experiences. Wurmser (1997) states, ". . . stimulants provide a sense of mastery, control, invulnerability and grandeur . . . the amphetamine effect serves as a defense against . . . general feelings of unworthiness and weakness."

Often, the environmental response to these changes is reinforcing. The user experiences himself as more extroverted, charming and desirable, with the perception that others feel and behave differently toward him. Specifical-ly, patients report that when they are high, other men are more attracted to them, thus confirming the sense of feeling sexier and more attractive. In this sense, both cocaine and "crystal" are drugs that must be understood in an intersubjective and interpersonal context, since their effects are perceived to be extraordinarily powerful on the subject (the user) and on the object. This impact is experienced both on internalized object representations as well as external ones, i.e., the real people in the addict's world. The impact on internalized object relations is reflected in the rapid evaporation of shame that results from critical or negating introjects, i.e., failure to live up to an ego ideal of desirable manliness and power. This transformation of self-experi-ence is often experienced by the drug user as "making" people find him more attractive, thus reinforcing the self-experience. In simpler language, confidence, and self-assurance are attractive qualities that result in greater success in finding a partner. This interpersonal phenomenon distinguishes these drugs from opiates, for example, which tend to promote social with-drawal accompanied by an inner sense of poetic grace and warmth, obviating the need for interactions with real people.

When sex is added to the stimulant experience, its meaning and value are heightened and transformed. If a sexual experience is combined with intrana-sal or smoked cocaine or crystal methamphetamine, powerful and reciprocal-ly enhancing experiences occur. Fears of rejection or overwhelming reactions to rejection are diminished. Internalized object relations that generate feel-ings of inadequacy or shame are eclipsed for a time, as the drug induced positive affects transiently alter internalized object relation. There emerges an internally experienced sense of approval and encouragement of the sense of entitlement. The drug-induced positive affects alter feelings regarding body adequacy, in turn increasing the drive and courage to seek sexual experiences. In short, doing these drugs makes it much easier to cruise for sex and make contact with another person.

Patients using stimulants report that pre-existing sexual anxieties are absent. The ordinary time frame for sex can radically change: having sex for 6-12 hours can become a realistic and predictable event. Users frequently report that crack and "crystal" facilitate participation in uninhibited, "over the top" sex, sometimes including sadomasochism, the use of dildoes or fistfucking in ways that seem wholly inaccessible without drugs. Some are able to enjoy anal sex only when using these stimulant drugs. Orgasm may be delayed, or even impossible to achieve. While these drugs may cause impotence ("crystal dick"), sildenafil (Viagra) is sometimes utilized to facilitate maintenance of an erection.

These combined sexual and drug experiences often occur in "sleazy" settings–bathhouses, bookstores, encounters with strangers, sex-and-drug hookups through the Internet, cruising the neighborhood or a bar. For some gay men, these "sleazy" qualities may contribute to the excitement as both the drug use and "pure sex" pursuit offer a transgressive thrill, i.e., "it's fun to be bad." However, this transgressive quality is not necessarily a major aspect of the gratification. Instead, the core desired experience is the apparently magical deliverance from inhibitions brought on by shame, feelings of inadequacy, self-fragmentation, internalized homophobia, anxiety, fragile ego states or dependent/counterdependent struggles into a predictably intense, sexual trance state of extended duration. The desirability of the drug/ sex experience is only heightened by its apparent controllability. Relationship problems, work related stress, fatigue, ordinary human limitations, loneliness, anxiety, depression are transiently banished and the user feels able to actually inhabit, however briefly, a grandiose self state: powerful, highly sexual, contained but uninhibited, intense, passionate, and aggressive. The drug has a profound effect on mood and behavior, which in turn alters the self-experience. There is a marked upsurge of self-idealization, feelings of omnipotence and grandiosity, self-acceptance, the expectation of acceptance by others embedded in a drug based euphoric state. There is a simultaneous experience of altered internalized object relations and an experience in the real world that (sometimes) enacts this fantasy: I am the powerful, admired, sexy man who is desired and accepted by a powerful and aroused Other/ Daddy. This is not merely an internal wish, but a wish that comes true: here is a perfect stranger, confirming the "reality" of the fantasy by participating in it with me, at least for right now. This does not make the fantasy into reality, but allows for a shared illusion, dependent on drug use for its intensity and for some men, the ability to inhabit play space of the shared illusion.

Some gay men use these stimulant drugs at infrequent intervals, and this tends to preserve more of the desired response. For others, the positive effects are so reinforcing that they are sought with increasing frequency and intake. For these men, the desired effects often become more and more elusive with continued use. As the love affair with the sex/drug experience reaches full bloom, the dark side (depression, paranoia, feeling "tweaked," compulsive, out of control use) emerges, as a result of the drugs' biologic and psychological sleight of hand. The relentless attempt to recapture the positive aspects of the experience ("chasing the high") usually leads to increased use, escalating negative consequences, physiological dependence and the stage of addiction in which use continues only to ward off the crashing despair of withdrawal. This depression is accentuated by the inevitable sadness of leaving the bathhouse, spent but lonely, ending an anonymous sexual encounter or being home alone.

DEVELOPMENTAL ISSUES

Several developmental themes emerge with frequency during the course of work with these men, which allow the therapist and ultimately the patient to appreciate the dynamic importance of the drug/sex addiction in maintaining a fragile or defective sense of self. Often, they report childhood experiences, common for some gay and proto-gay boys, of feelings of inadequacy, invisibility and difference, including an absence of athletic/physical recognition in grade school, high school and college. This commonly results in a sense of shame regarding both body and erotic feelings. Failure of parental and societal recognition and support of emerging sexuality generates self-imposed silence regarding sexual feelings and the inability to integrate sexuality into relationships and self-concept. These conditions combine to create an amalgam of shame, isolation, hopelessness, rage and sense of exclusion that is commonly labeled internalized homophobia. Even when there is compensatory narcissistic gratification through academic or professional achievements, the trauma and stigma of the invisible body, invisible self and negated sexuality remains painfully intense. This traumatic injury is felt concretely, in the body, and is experienced as factual and therefore as unhealable. The suffering is often experienced as truly being caused by insufficient muscularity, a face not handsome enough or a penis not large enough. Obsessive preoccupation with working out at the gym becomes the obvious solution with the twin hopes of becoming and attracting an idealized man. A profound sense of difference, abjection and nothingness is often coupled with interpersonal fear and self-loathing. This is "fixed" through belief in the ability to transform the self to become worthy of a relationship with a desirable Other who will mirror the grandiose, exciting, masculine self. This is concretized into (or onto) the surface and physical structure of the body. Weight training, management of body size through diet and steroid drugs and plastic surgery may become vital expressions of the drive to become visible, seen, noticed, admired, desired. Canarelli, Cole and Rizzuto movingly depict this process in their article, "Attention vs. Acceptance: Some Dynamic Issues in Gay Male Development." They describe the possible developmental paths through which the negation of the developing gay boy's desire leads to an impoverished sense of self and an exaggerated need for attention and validation in order to heal inner deadness.

Yet even the acquisition of a better or even superb body does not "fix" the archaic, unnoticed, invisible self. Its repair appears to be achieved, albeit temporarily, by successfully attracting and having sex with a virile man who both possesses *and* recognizes the virility and sexual desirability and desire of the subject. This transaction appears to be greatly facilitated by stimulant drug use. Patients report that they not only feel sexier and more able to engage in sex when using stimulant drugs, but that strangers on the street or in the bathhouse actually see them as sexier. When abstinent, the feelings of invisibility, asexuality and irrelevance return, and are experienced as "readable" by the external world, further validating the sense of the drug's power as real. When intoxicated on stimulants, all seems transformed, or at least potentially transformed, and the social contexts in which these drugs are used often enough make "dreams come true," if only for a while. This leads to the desire to repeat the experience again and again. For a while, at least, Cinderfella does achieve transformation. He changes from an unimpressive nothing into someone who gets to go to the ball, exhibit his new gown/body and dance with many dashing princes. He knows all the while that Midnight will come, when he will have to leave the ball and face the outside world. The body remains, but the subjective sense of its adequacy may fall precipitously. However, there is always the anticipation of another ball, another set of hunky princes, another evening of hot, sweaty dancing that awaits. Crystal or cocaine is the magic dust and a drug dealer is the fairy godfather that facilitates the transformation.

THE INITIAL CLINICAL PRESENTATION

When depression and fear of loss of control become overwhelming, individuals often seek or are referred for drug treatment. A sense of panic and shame accompany the experience of being unable to control one's use of sex and drugs. However, the patient is usually not committed to abstinence at this point, and any demand for it by a therapist is greatly feared/dreaded, although it may also be met with some relief. While the decision to seek evaluation for a drug problem certainly suggests a readiness to accept help, often the patient presents rationalizations that have protected him from acknowledging the progression of his addiction. These rationalizations might include: (1) comparing one's own drug use with the drug intake of heavier users, (2) recounting previous periods of abstinence in order to demonstrate strength of will, (3) condemning known abstinent individuals, and (4) isolating experiences from their greater context ("So I made a mistake. Next time, I'll stop sooner or use less."). This rationalization functions defensively to help the patient maintain the idea that the recent terrible experience, with its behavioral excesses and affective eruptions, represents the *beginning* of the presence of a substance use disorder. This reflects denial of the long-standing, deep attachment to the drug-sex experience. There is an understandable wish to go back to a prior pattern of use that appeared non-problematic.

It is useful for therapists to approach this phase of treatment with a mixture of psychoeducational and cognitive therapy techniques and a detailed inquiry into the drug history and subjective experience of drug use. This technique seeks to open up the patient's direct experience in both affective and behavioral terms. A valuable guide to this approach is *Psychotherapy of Cocaine Addiction–Entering the Interpersonal World of the Cocaine Addict,* by David Mark and Jeffrey Faude.

Traditional chemical dependency treatment techniques often suggest focusing exclusively on the negative experiences of drug use, concerned that accepting "romanticized" drug memories stirs up drug craving and fosters relapse. However, intense forms of resistance appear early and many patients are alienated by efforts to transform "good" experiences into "bad" ones. There are several problems with only emphasizing the negative aspects of the drug/sex experience. It implies that the therapist believes that the patient has been engaging in costly destructive behavior for no good reason, and is therefore foolish or deeply self-destructive. It short circuits the exploration of the profoundly important role of the sex/drug experience in altering self-states or self cohesion, or their role in transiently controlling painful affective states of loneliness and rejection. The detailed inquiry into drug experiences also can provide clues of co-morbid psychiatric disorders, guiding the use of psychotropic medication. If the therapist and patient examine experiences closely, the patient's initial idealizing report will often yield a more nuanced description with elements of obsession or loss of control, as well as post-intoxication depression, despair and suicidal ideation. These core elements need to be acknowledged if the patient is to change his relationship to drugs and sexuality.

This acknowledgement is, however, avoided because it portends the appearance of an overwhelming and terrifying loss: the stabilizing role that the drugs and sex play in maintaining psychic equilibrium. It may seem paradoxical that a destabilizing experience (such as a 12-hour drug and sex binge) is experienced as stabilizing. However, it is vital to explore this contradiction with the patient. Often patients need the therapist to acknowledge how wonderful some elements of drug use can be. If the therapist doesn't "get" this, the patient may fear that the therapist will not appreciate or understand what the impending loss will mean, that the loss is experienced as real, not illusory. As sexuality is also involved, a great deal is at stake. It is not just the affective and behavioral relationship with the drug and sex buddies that will be lost. Much worse is the threat to the patient's transient transformation into someone uninhibited and sexually successful. Patients are exquisitely sensitive to any hint of disapproval of the patterns of sexuality that they engage in, and respond with anger or withdrawal to any sense of therapist judgement. The therapist must appreciate, early on, the rigid narcissistic defenses the patient has needed and must recognize the compromised judgement and regressive defenses (denial and projection) with which the patient wards off intense shame and humiliation.

Another complication in the acknowledgement of the drug addiction is the question of sexual addiction, which patients often report with great fear and shame. The patterns are similar to those of drug addiction: loss of control, continued engagement in the behavior in spite of negative consequences, desire to stop with inability to do so, obsession with the experiences, intent to decrease frequency, etc. While the patient is in the stage of accepting the diagnosis of stimulant dependence, it is best to defer the definitive diagnosis of a sexual addiction. This is not because compulsive sexual behavior does not exist as a problem for some of these patients, but focusing on the sexual behavior distracts from the priority of this phase of treatment, the chemical addiction, and the sexual compulsivity may not persist in the state of drug abstinence. The goal of this part of the treatment is acceptance that any use of stimulants usually or invariably leads to extreme negative consequences, that sincere efforts to alter this pattern have failed, and that abstinence from stimulant drugs is necessary. It cannot be predicted that sexually compulsive behavior will persist in the context of abstinence from drugs. It often does not, although the loss of the very high level of sexual activity is usually experienced ambivalently, since sexual activity itself performs a vital function in affect management and self-stabilization. The drug induced sexual activity helps provide a grandiose sense of self, tenuously maintained in the face of poor affect tolerance and painful acknowledgement of limitations. The cognitive distortions seen in active drug addiction may lead the patient to believe that no other barrier will stand between them and overwhelming negative affects and self experiences except sex on drugs, and the threatened loss triggers a reactive protectiveness of the relationship with drugs and sex.

ESTABLISHMENT OF EARLY ABSTINENCE

The process of making a commitment to drug abstinence may take many months, and is often marked by brief episodes of abstinence alternating with return to active drug use. Just as patients dabble with drug use before becoming deeply attached to the experiences, experimentation with the thoughts and behaviors of abstinence often occurs before acceptance of the need for a basic change in the relationship with drugs and sex, and the readiness to make that commitment. Great anxiety and protest emerge at the loss of heightened sexuality, and this presages the core struggle of ongoing abstinence and sobriety.

It is common addiction treatment practice to explore the quality of the drug experiences, with the "discovery" that they weren't so great, that losing them isn't such a great loss and that sobriety offers ample compensatory pleasures. This occurs commonly with substance dependence syndromes that do not involve sex, and the pleasures and growth available in sobriety richly reward the efforts applied. This is often not the case with patients addicted to sex and drugs. In fact, the memories of drug-heightened sex become a challenge to progress as the patients eagerly hope for restitution of the powerful psychic effects of drug and sex experiences. They seek guidance on how to have sex that matches the previous intensity, or endure sexual experimentation in the "old places," becoming dismayed or disgusted by the environments or disappointed by the sex. The memories of drug and sex experiences make it even more difficult to explore inhibitions or anxieties that impair or limit sexual/romantic pleasure and satisfaction, since drugs were such an efficient, if short-term "magical" solution. The memories (often condensed into the self-state designated as "horniness") may function as a defense mechanism (grandiose self-idealization) that keeps anxiety, shame, or depressive feelings out of consciousness. A sense of anxiety and restlessness warn of a threat to self-cohesion and breakthrough of a self-experience of emptiness or invisibility, consciously experienced as the urge for rapid restitution of the idealized and sexualized masculine self. Hints of these "signal affects" often are transformed into a perceived "need to get high and get laid" that has an urgent, peremptory quality. This is an action-oriented, alloplastic response to perceived inner deadness. Sexual longing in the exposed state of abstinence may seem both vitally important and extremely anxiety provoking, because it triggers drug craving. Without stimulants, sexual experiences themselves may seem dull, lackluster, ordinary, or even impossible. Mourning and loss often alternate with denial and bargaining to find a way to go back to earlier days when the negative aspects of drug use seemed less problematic.

DOES ABSTINENCE FROM DRUGS REQUIRE CELIBACY?

Early in sobriety, sexual behavior can sometimes trigger intense craving, so traditional addiction treatment wisdom would advise sexual abstinence during early drug recovery. The patient will usually see this stance as a moralistic, prohibitive one that offers a confusing mixed signal regarding the role of pleasure and intimate contact. Is it possible to take a neutral, non-judgmental stance regarding sexual experience during this period that nonetheless offers support for early recovery? It is at this point that the fusion of sex and drugs is most exposed. One must admit that "over-the-top" sexual experiences will probably be inaccessible to the patient, at least for a while. There are two reasons for this: first, the direct brain effect of stimulant drugs on sex drive and intensity is gone. Thus, an intense sexual experience is difficult to access due to the withdrawal, caused by depletion of neurotransmitters involved. The second reason is that the pre-existing affects re-emerge, exaggerated both physiologically and psychologically, inhibiting the feelings of sexual ferocity that are sought. Is it advisable to suggest to the patient that super-aroused states, previously available only through drugs, can be found in some way, in sobriety? What is the optimal time to question the "packed" or multiply determined nature of the familiar assertion of "horniness"? These recurrent clinical questions raise the inevitable labeling of "good" versus "bad" kinds of sex. It is important to separate questions of the meaning of anonymous, "recreational" sex from drug use, even though they are fused in the patient's experience. The therapist must directly acknowledge the patients "right" to pursue the type of sexuality he chooses, as these are highly valued experiences, containing important, if fragmented, archaic self-object transferences that are not easily accessed in sobriety. Often, the sexuality during drug use is experienced as highly sensual, exciting, "animalistic," and greatly satisfying in a purely physical way. Sober sex is far more invaded by fluctuating internal states and fantasies. These may be distinctly anti-erotic, or at best, a dim version of the former intensity. It is precisely the banishment of these feelings, and the evocation of a grandiose, eroticized self-state that is part of the desired drug effects.

It is common for the patient to rightly assume the therapist privileges a more related, intimate type of sexuality, while also appreciating the exuberant delights that patients frequently report when describing their drug/sex experiences. There is often a broad range of countertransference reactions to these wild and ribald stories, including envy, nostalgia, excitement, and anxiety. Sexuality in the context of greater intimacy or a relationship may or may not be a conscious goal for the patient, and even if it is, he may find many very real obstacles to it, both within himself and in his familiar social milieu. Is the possibility of a deeply exciting and passionate sober sexuality for these patients realistic, or does their positive, repetitive response to drug/sex bespeak real limitations to this ever happening, the situation being made worse, biologically and psychologically, by the rapacious chemicals? From a clinical/philosophic point of view, do we assume that the use of drugs to achieve this state somehow renders the experience less real, counterfeit, or desperately compensatory? Does it stand in the place of a more "mature" use of sexuality? These forced binaries are themselves a result of thinking that is reductionistic. It is foolhardy to declare an experience as unreal, when the patient's direct knowledge declares otherwise. Since its occurrence, at a psychic level, requires extraordinary manipulation of affect and defense through drugs, it comes into existence through the prosthetic effects of the stimulants. It seems unlikely that an exact replica can be found in sobriety. However, the process of psychotherapy and recovery can reduce the demand for compensatory idealized self states through increased self acceptance and greater affect tolerance, which in turn lead to greater access to passion and abandon into sexuality.

THERAPEUTIC APPROACHES: TRANSFERENCE AND RESISTANCE

In early recovery, the appropriate goal is the exploration of the patient's ambivalence about abstinence, his achievement of it, and the re-establishment of abstinence in the event of relapse. It is a serious error to assume that abstinence is an unambivalent goal of the patient, even though he is knowingly in treatment that is based on it. It is a familiar, frustrating process for the therapist and patient alike when the therapist assumes the patient "knows" the "right" thing to do, then doesn't do it. Didactic approaches, moralization, gentle or combative threats or admonishments are rarely of any value. The patient may see the therapist as someone who wishes to control him and his use, punishing him for "being bad." He may overtly rebel against the sense of domination, calmly continuing to use while the therapist contains the anxiety and feeling of being out of control. The patient may alternatively submit to the therapist's "wishes," attempting to please and appease the voice of authority, all the while plotting a rebellion. The clinician's task in early recovery is to determine the type of therapeutic response that will explore these resistances and help the patient come to experience the commitment to abstinence as his own. The therapist may offer help by interpreting these resistances while demonstrating his own lack of need to control the patient.

Once the patient personally commits to abstinence, the therapist can intervene to simultaneously reduce the intensity of affects that trigger craving and relapse and support the expression and containment of emergent self-states. It is crucial to reframe these emergent states as valuable, albeit uncomfortable. It can be necessary to explicitly maintain and express the belief that a growing tolerance for these states is necessary for their transformation.

The transference/countertransference processes seen in the treatment of drug addiction are well described by Kaufman (1992) and Imhof, Hirsch and Terenzi (1984). Of particular interest is the phenomenon of the patient's use of the therapist as a drug substitute. This often shows itself first through a countertransference experience of being in a narrow or collapsed space with little therapeutic power or magic dust to sprinkle that would make things feel better quickly. This represents the experience elicited by the patient's unconscious engagement with the therapist as a wished for drug substitute. At these times, there is intense pressure to offer hope or proof to the patient that the move from active drug use to sobriety is "worth it." The therapist becomes the spokesman for sobriety, and feels responsible for "selling it." One often sees much balancing and weighing of the positive and negative consequences of drug use compared with skepticism regarding the likelihood of "getting" anything from the sobriety that will feel good. Attempts to convince the patient of the value of sobriety are futile, since this misses the fear being expressed. It is more valuable for the therapist to hold and contain these fears, facilitating the capacity to tolerate these inner states. Verbalization of these affects and emergent self-states by the therapist, leading to the patient's experience of being held and cared for can gradually increase the tolerance for them. This occurs both for the patient and therapist, who may identify with the patient's insistent demand for results and tools as analogous to his own experience of therapeutic invisibility and lack of a tool big enough for this job.

The patient's ambivalent relationship with sobriety can be externalized into the therapist and expressed in the transference in other ways. He may see the therapist as a crusader for abstinence, a moralizing goody-goody who disapproves of drugs and wild sex. The patient then becomes the rebellious, Dionisian pleasure seeker, escaping from external demands to "be good," angrily overthrowing "the Law." In this way, the struggle with abstinence is externalized. Tension is reduced because the conflict is experienced as a struggle between the "wishes" of the therapist and the patient. Some patients feel controlled by fear of disappointing the therapist, having to endure the anticipated withdrawal, disapproval or scorn if he relapses due to lack of "will power" or inner strength, or as proof of his lack of need for help. In this situation, the drug use may function both as a rebellion against that constraint (abstaining out of fear of disapproval or loss of love) and an eraser of the guilt for the wish to destroy the therapist's perceived power or goodness. For other patients, the drug/sex relapse may function as a chemical solution for shame at failure to be "strong willed" enough to not need drugs and/or drug treatment, i.e., as a person with intense needs. Under the pressure of drug craving, the patient may perceive that he needs help (perhaps a great deal of it) in order to stay sober, but can get high on his own, thus repudiating the need for an Other and bolstering omnipotent defenses. This is a common paradox: relapse both demonstrates the failure of willpower, but chemically reinforces the illusion of self-sufficiency and omnipotence over emotional states.

Another common transference configuration is the patient's expressed belief that the therapist cannot really understand and accept the importance of sexuality to this particular patient. This dynamic is often accompanied by fantasies of the therapist leading a tranquil, "boring" life of gay domestic tranquillity proudly enjoying "opera tickets, a two bedroom apartment and regular attendance at the 26th Street antiques market." The patient may experience a need to see the therapist in a desexualized way, and this may serve several functions. He may feel that therapeutic events need to take place in a setting devoid of sexual feelings, contributing to a feeling of safety and protection. Sessions may need to be free of the treacherous explicit competitiveness and sexuality that can evoke shame and the experience of invisibility as well as competitiveness. As well, the attribution to the therapist of a bland, desexualized life may represent a projection of the patient's fears or wishes about himself. A similar pattern is the disavowal of any sexual or sexualized aspects of the therapeutic relationship, with the wish to preserve the treatment relationship as one free of that particular danger/excitement, or at least the explicit discussion of it, as if it represents something antithetical to the psychotherapy process. This seems to point to the patient's awareness of the dissociative and essentially conservative nature of his drug fueled sexuality, and his need to maintain a split between sexuality and personal growth, intimacy, empathic engagement and safety from exploitation.

The patient may at times, desire the therapist to contain these prohibiting positions regarding sexuality, perhaps as a projective identification of internalized objects who were silent and negating of his sexuality. He may fear admitting his lack of attraction to the therapist, concerned that this will be terribly hurtful or insulting. This reveals a projected aspect of his own traumatic experience of being desexualized through denial of emergent sexuality in childhood and adolescence, and the present day feeling of being invisible in the harsh competitiveness of the gay drug/sex subculture. Alternatively, sexual attraction between the therapist and patient may interfere with the patient's feeling of trust and safety. One patient informed me that a previous therapist had revealed that he found the patient sexually attractive. The patient ended the treatment soon after, because he didn't believe anyone experiencing sexual feelings toward him could also want to help him. I was instructed not to have such feelings toward him, while simultaneously being told of years of bodybuilding, steroids, plastic surgery and self-development that he had devoted to making himself attractive to gay men. He had projected into me the conflicted boy, admonished not to get excited while being shown exciting things. In his fantasy, he struggled to possess the overt and observed sexuality. Clearly, I was not to have any, or if I did, I was supposed to suppress and contain it, as he had had to do in his childhood. This projection alternated with painful moments of experiencing himself as unattractive, thin, and invisible, anxiously asking me if I noticed subtle changes in his muscularity or facial features.

RELAPSE FANTASIES

Relapse fantasies are a common occurrence in the long-term treatment of addictive disorders. There is a growing urgency that the patient will relapse if "something isn't done." There is an experience of life and the therapy as distinctly unexciting, possessing little, if any, of the hot, powerful stuff that is available at the bathhouse or from a drug dealer. Therapy is experienced as insufficiently stimulating and frustrating in its interiority. Its explicit privileging of verbal expression of affect, especially self-experiences with painful affect, rather than narcissistic and hypomanic acting out defenses, may begin to feel unuseful or even incomprehensible to the patient. The patient may pit active drug use against sobriety in direct competition, challenging the therapist to convince him that recovery is "better." Countertransference reactions include feelings of defensiveness of psychotherapy itself, with a compensatory wish to find a way to excite the patient about the journey of self-discovery, along with anger or hopelessness in response to the patient's devaluation and concreteness. If the therapy itself is regarded as a drug substitute, an antidote to craving itself, it is seen as falling short. The persistence of this ambivalence can lead to consideration of termination. A growing weariness in the patient (and sometimes the therapist) often precedes a relapse. The patient will report increasing drug obsession, growing doubt about "changing" and boredom. The relapse, if it occurs, finally resolves the obsession about whether or not to return to active drug use.

This brings the therapy to a particular kind of dilemma. Certainly, patient, calm inquiry into the circumstances of the relapse is indicated, unless life threatening circumstances require a more active approach. Re-teaching the "how's" of abstinence is of little use here, since the problem usually lies not so much with *how* to maintain abstinence, as it does with the question of *why*. On some occasions, relapses are presented as largely unpleasant, anxiety ridden and not at all reinforcing. Most times, the period of abstinence serves to set the stage, physiologically, for a highly positive initial return to familiar territory, filled with the ecstatic, "over-the-top" experiences that were sought, even if return of obsession, loss of control and marked affective dysregulation are the price to pay. The problems inherent in active drug use seem to pose less of a problem than do those that result from living outside it. Detailed inquiry into the experience often proves to be difficult, and the sexual experiences tend to be conveyed in a stereotyped way–the hotness of the man, the hotness of the sex, its duration and the number of partners. Big, embarrassed, goofy grins and excited affect usually accompany these stories. The longing for a pure Kohutian moment of mirroring is palpable, along with fear of disapproval or shame. The internal experience remains largely unarticulated, not readily accessible for exploration, especially in regard to the use of a sexual partner as a source of transient identification, self-stabilization against painful or frightening affect or foundering sense of self-cohesion. A common explanation that is offered is simply: "I was horny." Responding with the notion that such an explanation is lacking feels vaguely insulting and suspect to the patient. Wurmser (1997) refers to this process as "hyposymbolization," a curtailed ability to translate feelings into symbolic language, with a shift toward a more somatic or action oriented expression.

A common patient fear is that the therapist will criticize the patient's sexuality, drug use (or both), as depraved, needy, shameful. At times, there is the sense that the patient is trying to seduce the therapist. The seduction, however, is not so much into sexual arousal, but rather into believing in the validity and even the irreplaceable nature of the drug/sex experience, a kind of invitation away from the grim tasks of therapy.

It is interesting that some patients often wish for the therapist to have some experiences with the drugs in question in order to understand the difficulty of abstinence, but not too much experience. It seems important that the drug use be a part of the therapist's past, but not his present. This may be an expression of longing for the wished for gay father who can be loving, containing and understanding of intense homoerotic desire, while being available to control overstimulation and to provide safety from wishes that feel out of control or self destructive. The transference can reflect multiple identifications of the patient: the wish to be an uncloseted, confident adult gay man with "gay" desires and experiences and an excited goody-goody bystander who is intrigued by the rapacious sexual outlaw. The patient wishes for the therapist to help him integrate these disparate identities. There is pressure to show how life can be exciting in sobriety. Sobriety for the patient becomes a dreary foreign land, to which he feels exiled, sent away from the marvelous party by his own doing, and resenting the look of the new landscape. He wonders if the therapist's life is one worth identifying with.

SUMMING UP

It is particularly difficult to find a single valence for drug fueled sexuality, and to differentiate its misuse in an addiction process from its role as a response to the internalized homophobic and antisexual biases we are all subject to. Certainly, there are many ways to live as a gay man, but if drug use is experienced as vital to the uninhibited expression of one's "true" gay identity, can abstinence occur without a profound revision of such an identity? Is there a stable abstinence from drugs that is not coupled with the privileging of calmer, safer, cozier sexuality? Certainly, in theory, but it's not an easy place to get to when anxiety, feelings of invisibility and disappointing sexual experiences become overwhelming. Some patients in recovery from drug addiction find a profound positive change in their capacity for intimacy and their ability to maintain a relationship. Yet they may still have moments of nostalgic longing for their "basic (old) program: get drunk, get high, get laid." A stable path toward sustained abstinence occurs when multiple aspects of a patient's life improve so clearly as a result of recovery that the idea of returning to drug use is not a realistic consideration, even under the pressure of euphoric recall of drug/sex experiences. These improvements are usually both in the personal, relational world as well as the world of work and avocations. In this situation, changes in sexuality are usually accepted and explored, with some ambivalent nostalgia. Commonly, patients say they don't regret having had a drug/sex addiction, but are grateful that they've escaped from it with most of their life intact.

There are several important processes that significantly contribute to positive outcomes in the treatment of these men. The establishment of a stable, containing treatment setting in which to examine the relationship with stimulant drugs and sex can lead to the reduction in defenses against awareness of the negative consequences of the addiction. This stabilizes recovery. Clarification and explication of the defenses of denial, minimization, projection, splitting, *as applied to the relationship with the drug itself*, can lead to greater persistence of the experienced need for abstinence and thus the patient is able to withstand greater storms of craving and longing. Patients also find in sobriety, inevitably, a greater acceptance of their interior world, regardless of the kind of character structure that underlay the heightened receptivity to the drug experience in the first place. Abstinence and recovery in these patients is almost always accompanied by a moving sense of reacquaintance or rediscovery of their former self, however troubled it may have felt. The strengths of the pre-addiction self are recognized and reappreciated once outside the invisible grasp of the addictive process. And the sex? Well, each man returns to his own world, returned to the more ordinary struggles for intimacy and sexual expression that have challenged us for millennia.

REFERENCES

Canarelli, Joseph, Cole, Gilbert and Rizzuto, Charles (1998), Attention vs. Acceptance: Some Dynamic Issues in Gay Male Development. *Gender and Psychoanalysis: An Interdisciplinary Journal*, Vol. 4: No. 1: 47-70.

Dodes, Lance (1990), Addiction, Helplessness and Narcissistic Rage. *Psychoanalytic Quarterly*, LIX: 398-419.

Imhof, John, Hirsch, Robert and Terenzi, Richard (1984), Countertransferential and Attitudinal Considerations in the Treatment of Drug Abuse and Addiction. *The Journal of Substance Abuse Treatment*, Vol. 1: 21-30.

Johnson, Brian (1999), Three Perspectives on Addiction. *Journal of the American Psychoanalytic Association*, Vol. 47: 3, pp. 791-815.

Khantzian, Edward (1995), Self-Regulation Vulnerabilities in Substance Abusers: Treatment Implications. In *The Psychology and Treatment of Addictive Behavior*, ed. Scott Dowling. Madison: International Universities Press, pp. 17-41.

Khantzian, Edward (1997), The Self-Medication Hypotheses of Addictive Disorders: Focus on Heroin and Cocaine Dependence. In *Essential Papers On Addiction*, ed. Daniel Yalisove. New York: New York University Press, pp. 429-440.

Kaufman, Edward (1992), Countertransference and Other Mutually Interactive Aspects of Psychotherapy with Substance Abusers. *The American Journal on Addictions*, Vol.1: No. 3: pp. 185-202.

Krystal, Henry (1997), Self-Representation and the Capacity for Self-Care. In *Essential Papers on Addiction*, ed. Daniel Yalisove. New York: New York University Press, pp. 109-146.

Ling, Walter, Los Angeles Addiction Research Consortium (1998), Proceedings of Ninth Annual Meeting and Symposium of the American Academy of Addiction Psychiatry, p. 13.

Mark, David and Faude, Jeffrey (1997), *Psychotherapy of Cocaine Addiction: Entering the Interpersonal World of the Cocaine Addict*. Northvale, New Jersey: Jason Aronson, Inc.

Morgenstern, Leeds (1993), Contemporary Psychoanalytic Theories of Substance Abuse: A Disorder in Search of a Paradigm," *Psychotherapy*, Vol. 30, No. 2, pp. 194-206.

Wallace, John (1978), The Dangers of Psychotherapy in the Treatment of Alcoholism. In *Practical Approaches to Alcoholism Psychotherapy*, ed. Zimberg, Sheldon, Wallace, John and Blume, Sheila G., New York: Plenum Press.

Wurmser, Leon (1995), Compulsiveness and Conflict: The Distinction between Description and Explanation in the Treatment of Addictive Behavior. In *The Psychology and Treatment of Addictive Behavior*, ed. Scott Dowling, Madison: International University Press, pp. 43-64.

Wurmser, Leon (1997), Psychoanalytic Considerations of the Etiology of Compulsive Drug Use. In *Essential Papers on Addiction*, ed. Daniel Yalisove, New York City: New York University Press, pp. 87-108.

Wurmser, Leon (1987), Flight from Conscience: Experiences with the Psychoanalytic Treatment of Compulsive Drug Abusers: Part One: Dynamic Sequences Underlying Compulsive Drug Use; Part Two: Dynamic and Therapeutic Conclusions from the Experiences with Psychoanalysis of Drug Users. *Journal of Substance Abuse Treatment*, Vol. 4. pp. 157-179.

Zimberg, Sheldon, Wallace, John and Blume, Sheila G. (1978), *Practical Approaches to Alcoholism Psychotherapy*, New York: Plenum Press.

Psychoanalytic and Behavioral Approaches to Drug-Related Sexual Risk Taking: A Preliminary Conceptual and Clinical Integration

David G. Ostrow, MD, PhD
R. Dennis Shelby, PhD

SUMMARY. The topic of substance abuse among gay and bisexual men is of intense topical interest precisely because of the demonstrated co-occurrence of "recreational" substance use and HIV infection among gay/bisexual men. With the discovery of the Human Immunodeficiency Virus Type-I (HIV), it has been consistently shown that both prevalent and incident HIV infections are significantly associated with a history of substance use or abuse. In an attempt to integrate both cognitive-behavioral models and psychoanalytical understandings of our drug using/sexual risk-taking patients, the authors have engaged in the exchange of ideas and case reports over the past several years. This paper summarizes the results of those exchanges and utilizes two clinical case examples as the basis for identifying the utility of an integrated psychoanalytical and behavioral approach to clinical conceptualization and treatment. *[Article copies available for a fee from The Haworth Document Delivery Service: 1-800-342-9678. E-mail address: <getinfo@haworthpress inc.com> Website: <http://www.HaworthPress.com>]*

Dr. David G. Ostrow is Chief of Addiction Medicine Program and Professor of Psychiatry and Behavioral Neurosciences, Loyola University School of Medicine. Dr. R. Dennis Shelby is affiliated with the Institute for Clinical Social Work and is a Candidate, Chicago Institute for Psychanalysis.

Address correspondence to: Dr. David G. Ostrow, Professor, Psychiatry and Behavioral Neurosciences, Chief, Loyola Addiction Medicine Program (LAMP), Loyola University Medical School, 2160 South First Avenue, Building 54, Room 157, Maywood, IL 60153 (E-mail: dostro1@luc.edu).

[Haworth co-indexing entry note]: "Psychoanalytic and Behavioral Approaches to Drug-Related Sexual Risk Taking: A Preliminary Conceptual and Clinical Integration." Ostrow, David G., and R. Dennis Shelby. Co-published simultaneously in *Journal of Gay & Lesbian Psychotherapy* (The Haworth Medical Press, an imprint of The Haworth Press, Inc.) Vol. 3, No. 3/4, 2000, pp. 123-139; and: *Addictions in the Gay and Lesbian Community* (ed: Jeffrey R. Guss, and Jack Drescher) The Haworth Medical Press, an imprint of The Haworth Press, Inc., 2000, pp. 123-139. Single or multiple copies of this article are available from The Haworth Document Delivery Service [1-800-342-9678, 9:00 a.m. - 5:00 p.m. (EST). E-mail address: getinfo@haworthpressinc.com].

© 2000 by The Haworth Press, Inc. All rights reserved.

KEYWORDS. Drug use, homosexuality, cognitive-behavioral treatments, psychoanalytical treatments, HIV-risk, escape coping, sex-drug use

INTRODUCTION

The topic of substance abuse among gay and bisexual men being addressed is of intense topical interest precisely because of the demonstrated co-occurrence of "recreational" substance use and HIV infection among gay/bisexual men (Ostrow, 2000). Few studies have looked at the rates and problematic aspects of substance use/abuse among gay/bisexual men and fewer have dealt with the associated sexual behavior issues before the discovery in 1981 of *acquired immunodeficiency syndrome* (AIDS) among otherwise healthy gay men (CSAP, 1994). By 1984, the senior author, working with data from the Multicenter AIDS Cohort Study (the MACS; Ostrow et al., 1990), and Ronald Stall, working with the San Francisco Men's Health Study (the SFMHS; Stall et al., 1986), simultaneously observed that men reporting substance use were more likely to be engaging in unprotected anal intercourse (UAI) and were less likely to reduce their risk if they continued using substances. With the discovery of the Human Immunodeficiency Virus Type-I (HIV), it has been consistently shown that both prevalent and incident HIV infection is significantly associated with a history of substance use or abuse (Ostrow et al., 1995; Chesney, Barrett and Stall, 1998; Stall and Purcell, 2000).

Since there are no credible reasons that drug use *per se* can cause AIDS but rather is likely to be a behavioral marker for high risk sexual activity and/or a co-factor in HIV transmission (Watson, 1990), the search for causal mechanism(s) responsible for these associations takes on added importance for primary and secondary AIDS prevention among gay men. As outlined in one of the earliest papers on this topic (Stall et al., 1986), the behavioral connections between substance use and UAI among gay men can be conceptualized as belonging to four general categories, each having particular importance for HIV/AIDS prevention:

1. Direct "pharmacological" actions of substances which increase sexual desires or the intensity of the sexual experience, otherwise thought of as aphrodisiacs (*direct drug action models*)
2. Indirectly, by decreasing cognitive awareness of the risks involved or leading to the ineffective use of safer sex measures, such as the incorrect use of condoms or non-compatible oil-based lubricants (*cognitive inhibition models*)
3. Indirectly, through the presence of a common underlying vulnerability, such as high sensation seeking, sexual compulsivity or risk-taking per-

sonality traits, that may be associated with both substance use and sexual risk taking (*common underlying vulnerability models*)

4. Variations and various combinations on the above (*mixed effects models*). In particular, we have recently put forth a theory that the strategic use of drugs to escape cognitive inhibitions to unprotected sex may underlie the use of drugs in the sexual context for men who are aware of the risks involved in mixing sex and drugs but wish to experience the added intimacy and pleasure that anal sex without a condom can provide (the escape model, labeled the "AIM Model," Ostrow & McKirnan 1997; McKirnan, Ostrow & Hope, 1996).

In addition, plausible *biological co-factor models* include local drying or irritation of mucosal membranes (as is known to occur with crack cocaine and marijuana smoking), vasodilatation (volatile nitrite use), and acute immunosuppressive effects of volatile nitrite inhalation (Dax et al., 1991).

As useful as these models might be for the design and interpretation of behavioral research studies, their focus on the cognitive level of sexual behavior, decision making in the dyadic sexual context, and the conscious choices that individuals make when presented with drug use and sexual opportunities leaves much to be desired in the psychotherapeutic setting. As elegantly discussed by Dr. Walter Odets (Odets, 1994) and others, cognitive-behavioral explanations are only one dimension of the complex of conscious and unconscious motivations to engage in risky behaviors observed among many gay and bisexual men seen in therapy. In an attempt to integrate both cognitive-behavioral models and psychoanalytical understandings of our drug using/sexual risk-taking patients, the authors have engaged in the exchange of ideas and case reports over the past several years. This paper summarizes the results of those exchanges and utilizes two clinical case examples as the basis for identifying the utility of an integrated approach to clinical conceptualization and treatment. In addition, where there are conflicting interpretations of the case material from the two conceptual frameworks, these are pointed out and discussed in terms of the challenges which may lie ahead for psychotherapy and prevention work with substance using gay men. Clinical intervention usually entails more variables than any single research study or theoretical model can consider. Different clinical models lend themselves to different populations, settings and individual patient psychopathologies. In these days of diminishing treatment resources, both public and private, clinicians should avail themselves of a range of intervention models. The ultimate issue is not theoretical superiority, rather theoretical and treatment model utility given the population, setting and resources.

CASE STUDY 1 AND PSYCHOANALYTICAL INTERPRETATION

Case Study 1: Mr. A was a tall, sturdily built 26-y/o man. He had a large black moustache and piercing blue eyes. He was employed as a waiter in a restaurant that catered to an often rowdy after-hours crowd in a neighborhood where many heterosexual bars were located. Mr. A looked more like a construction laborer than a waiter. In the course of sessions he would often become overwhelmed and be unable to speak. He never missed a session in 2 years, but for the first year, would often be unable to talk for most of the hour.

PRESENTING COMPLAINTS

Mr. A was referred by his physician after several months of somatic complaints, and what were described as hysterical office visits during which Mr. A would come in worried that he had contracted an STD and demand testing. The physician could never ascertain exactly what sexual activity Mr. A had engaged in, as Mr. A would become anxious, overwhelmed and be unable to speak when asked about his activities. Mr. A consistently refused HIV testing, relating that he understood safer sex guidelines, but hinted that he was not always following them.

COURSE OF TREATMENT

Mr. A was both engaging and appeared terrified. Obtaining a history and general ideas about his concerns was slow and arduous for both of us. When asked questions, Mr. A would think for a while then quickly blurt out the answers. He was certain that he had contracted HIV but could not tolerate the idea of being tested. He reported that he was repeatedly overwhelmed at work, mixing up food orders, or dropping trays of food. While working he felt that something bad was about to happen and it usually did. In general, Mr. A seemed determined to convince me that he was incompetent. He had accumulated considerable credits in various community colleges, but was unable to decide on a degree or general course for his life. He felt stuck in the waiting job, but unable to decide what he wanted to do in the long term. He was genuinely puzzled when I offered that his current preoccupation with STDs must mean something in terms of what he was going through at this stage in his life, his fear of HIV, and feelings about himself and men.

Slowly a sketch of Mr. A's history emerged. He was the youngest of a sibship of three. He grew up in a large town just outside of Chicago. Parents divorced early on, he was raised primarily by his grandmother while mother worked and was dating one man after another. He maintained sporadic contact with both parents; his grandmother was alive and well and continued to be a source of support. When asked about early memories, he became overwhelmed and related that he had recurring dreams of being chased home from school almost daily by bullies.

Just as Mr. A appeared more comfortable and settled into treatment, the sessions became quite rocky. He would often sit for long periods, appearing on the verge of being overwhelmed, then blurt out what was troubling him. At times, it was an upsetting incident at work that left him flooded with feelings of incompetence. At other times it was related to the deepening of the transference and painful feelings about himself that he was trying to bring into the treatment. Mr. A reported frequent episodes of becoming overwhelmed at work, mixing up orders, becoming tongue-tied with his often intoxicated customers. In his sessions, with a great deal of encouragement, he would slowly tell me what had happened. Initially, he saw no relationship between what occurred, his self-states, or that these incidents may mean something. One day he related that he was waiting on a group of people, one of the drunken men called him a "faggot." The customer's girlfriend proceeded to scold the man for his behavior. Mr. A found this especially humiliating in that he felt he should be able to standup for himself, not rely on a girl. He then began to realize that working around rowdy straight men who were intoxicated reminded him of the repeated assaults and humiliations he encountered as a child from the neighborhood bullies. Later he recalled the many drunken fights between his parents, before the divorce and his father's exit from the home.

As the transference deepened, Mr. A struggled to bring into the treatment his painful sense of gender defectiveness. Initially he interpreted my neutrality and inquisitiveness as not believing him. One day he screamed, "Don't you get it? I am a sissy! A big sissy! I sew fringe on lampshades and paint flower pots to look like Wedgwood!" Once Mr. A felt that I could accept his feelings of defectiveness and incompetence, he was better able to discuss his difficulties with men and sex. He was terrified of meeting men. In a bar he would become overwhelmed, hide in a corner and drink. If someone did approach him, he would be unable to hold a conversation. Mr. A tended to seek out sexual encounters in the baths or bookstores after a frustrating night in the bars. He was usually intoxicated by that time, and if he could afford it, would use cocaine before going out to the bars and throughout the evening. By the time he ended up in the baths or bookstores he was acutely intoxicated and frustrated and would let his partners do whatever they wanted to him, or do to them whatever they wanted him to do to them. Gradually he was able to relate that he did this so he would not have to talk. He felt safer sex required talking, and if he talked, his partners would find out that he was a sissy and reject him. He felt horribly guilty and ashamed each time he ingested semen or engaged in passive anal intercourse without a condom. To say "No" risked being rejected and/or called a sissy.

Mr. A's preoccupation with contracting STDs diminished as did the emergency calls to his physician as he became more comfortable in the treatment relationship. As the treatment progressed, his presentation became less volatile. Disrupting events were more easily recognizable and interpreted. He managed to go out on a few dates, and discovered that negotiating safer sex boundaries was not that dangerous after all. He also discovered that when out for dinner and a movie, neither he or his partners drank as much, if at all. Initially he was quite aware of the newness of not using alcohol and drugs and often fought off considerable anxiety during his early attempts to date, rather than engage men in anonymous sex. Mr. A was able to discuss the anxiety he felt during longer extended sessions of sexuality that occurred in the bedroom versus the bathhouse, and also that he was beginning to enjoy sex more. Eventually he was able to relate that the best part was sleeping with a man afterwards. In tears, he related that what he really wanted was the sense of comfort and security of the extended contact of sleeping and cuddling after sex, not just sex. This too he felt was a sign of weakness, not a reasonable human longing. To his surprise, his partners seemed to want that also, and they rarely left after a sexual encounter, unlike his experience in the baths or bookstores. Mr. A was genuinely moved that men would want to spend time with him after sex, not just during fleeting anonymous encounters.

As the treatment progressed, Mr. A brought in a fantasy that had sustained him in childhood. In his desk at school was a magic chair. He could sit on it and fly around the schoolroom. When distressed after the incident with the bullies at school, he would daydream about dazzling his classmates with his flying chair. Unfortunately, his teachers would become frustrated by his "daydreaming" and publicly humiliate him for not paying attention. Concurrently Mr. A began to let me see his many areas of competence. He was quite organized with his monetary affairs and had saved a considerable sum should he return to school. He had an extensive social circle, and he would often cook elaborate holiday dinners for his friends. He had excelled in French, and had taken every French class offered in high school and the many community colleges he attended.

The final phase of the treatment saw Mr. A enrolling in college to finish a teaching degree in French. He related that he had always wanted to do this, but was afraid of standing in front of a class for fear of ridicule. He also began planning a trip to a French speaking Canadian city. Many hours were spent listening to his planning efforts, and his discovering just how much he enjoyed learning, and traveling. There were many glitches in planning the trip, but this time he appeared to be viewing my presence as reassuring rather than threatening. Each problem with the trip initially met with distress, but then a solution was found. Traveling too, had scared him, as he feared getting lost, or something bad happening should he venture too far from his home. The treatment wound down as Mr. A completed several semesters with good grades, negotiated his trip with ease, and tested negative for HIV.

DISCUSSION

In approaching the topic of drug use during sexual activity from a psychoanalytic perspective, we must begin with the central hypothesis of psychoanalysis: the vast majority of mental activity is unconscious. This perspective leads to questions regarding the unconscious, or pre-conscious awareness for the motivations to use psychoactive drugs while seeking out or engaging in sexual encounters. It also leads to questions regarding the structure of the individual psyche in terms of conflicts, vulnerabilities, defenses employed to manage conflicts and vulnerabilities and ultimately what is sought after in a sexual encounter. In the context of the clinical setting, we must also consider the therapeutic alliance, and the transferences.

Sexuality has always been an integral aspect of psychoanalytic theories. From the beginning Freud implicated sexuality in the etiology of hysteria (Freud 1896). In the Three Essays on the Theory of Sexuality (1905) Freud discussed the power of the sexual drives and began to offer a more complex theory of the role of sexuality in mental life in general. A central aspect of this effort was to offer explanations for why people did seemingly odd things involving sexual activity that were completely at odds with their day to day functioning. There has been an unfortunate tendency to read the Three Essays as a *Psychopathia Sexualis*. May (1995) points out that the work can also be understood as a treatise on the many possibilities of the sexual mind. Clearly Freud's endpoint was heterosexual genital intercourse, but he did not view heterosexuality as a "given." Rather it was the result of complex developmental and intrapsychic factors.

The "right" of individuals to engage in sexual activity that places them at risk for infection with the HIV virus is a topic of much heated debate. "Rights" aside, many of us consider it somewhat odd that persons would engage in risky behavior if they are HIV negative. As stated above, research has consistently indicated that recreational drugs play a role in sexual activities that place the individual at greatest risk for HIV/STD infection. This leads one to wonder what is the function of the drug for the person using it during sexual encounters as well as what is the function of the sexual activity?

Freud's initial conceptualization of perversion as relating to the (unconscious) choice of the sexual object (person) and fetish (the lingering over an intermediate area, e.g., hair, feet, etc.) moved to the background as theorists focused on some aspect of the Oedipal conflict being played out in the course of sexuality. Unfortunately, the term perversion came to be used for any sexual activity outside the male/female missionary position "norm." Stoller (1975) emphasized the role of rage in esoteric sexual behavior and offered that for some people sexual activity was an effort to turn a humiliation into a triumph. In recent years the focus has shifted to sexualization: the defensive use of sexuality and the role of *affects* rather than drives and conflict. In other words, sexuality is used as a defense to manage a conflict, inhibition, or self-deficit.

Kohut's self psychology has turned our attention to the needs, structural vulnerabilities deficits in the self versus the drive model which emphasized forces seeking expression and forces seeking to repress those very forces. In the self-psychology model, the emphasis shifts to the self striving for coherence and sustaining relations with others and vulnerabilities that interfere with these needs. The role of sexuality in managing deficits and affects becomes the focus. Kohut (1971) offered that frantic, sexualized activities were often efforts to forestall further fragmentation of the self. Goldberg (1972) discussed the role of sexuality in managing distressed affects. More elaborate formulations were offered (Goldberg, 1995) to account for the complexity of some forms of sexual behavior and have been their role in the larger structure of the self. A central point of Goldberg's is the use of disavowal as a defense in some forms of sexual behavior. Disavowal entails the ignoring of "meaning" or a piece of "reality" and is a very different defense than denial, which pertains to the management of affects. For some individuals, sexuality, sexualization and disavowal become central "emergency measures" for managing distressing affects. The very behavior that puts some people at risk for HIV infection, legal consequences or financial ruin is the very activity employed to manage a distressed self.

When thinking about the role of recreational drugs in sexual activity from the psychoanalytic perspective, *three* distinctly different possibilities are evident: (1) the management of an inhibition, (2) efforts to express a sexual fantasy, and (3) efforts to disavow a problematic piece of reality. Goldberg (1995) and Tolpin (1997) have both discussed how sexuality is an activity of a healthy robust self. However a vulnerable self may be threatened by such an intense engagement with another person. Hence recreational drugs may be used to manage anxiety as the person attempts to engage another human being. (This conceptualization would have direct analogies to the cognitive-behavioral model of *direct aphrodisiac effects*, as aphrodisiacs are often seen as acting by reducing the inhibitory anxiety associated with the sexual act.) Freud's original definition of inhibition was that it reflected an "inhibition of an ego function" (1926). A socially inhibited person may use drugs that temporarily minimize anxiety and vulnerability in order to engage another person. In the second area, some sexual fantasies, such as sadistic or masochistic fantasies, may require a dampening down of the observing ego in order to let a fantasy (that is usually confined to masturbation) play out with another person(s) (in analogy to the *escape model* discussed above). Specific recreational drugs such as poppers and crystal are often employed as integral components of more adventurous activities such as "fist fucking" and bathhouse sex. While the role of poppers (volatile nitrites) is often discussed in relation to its ability to relax the anal sphincter, observation in the clinical setting indicates that this and other drugs also enhance and focus sexual fantasy (for example many men use poppers in masturbation that does not involve anal stimulation). In the third area, drugs may be employed to ignore aspects of reality (disavowal), such as the pain associated with an activity, the dangerous nature of the activity, that the partner is a "player, not the real thing" or the reality that a certain activity has been closely associated with HIV infection, again suggesting analogies to the *cognitive escape model.*

These are not mutually exclusive and one often observes a mixture, as in the *mixed affects models* of behavioral research. In the first the self is vulnerable and needs the drug to manage the seeming intimacy of a sexual encounter. In the second, the self is striving to express a sexual fantasy and let it "take over" and in the third, the self ignores reality in order to let the fantasy lead the way. In this perspective it is often useful to think in terms of the metaphor of the fantasy that drives the activity–what is the person attempting to achieve via the activity, and what is the self state of the person before and after they engage in the activity? This approach will help the therapist to remain focused on the sexual behavior in the context of the dynamic meaning, structural capacities and cognitive awareness of the self. In this way the therapist is forced to think about the patient's problematic behavior from a combined cognitive and psychoanalytical perspective from the earliest stage of the treatment, particularly with fragile patients for whom focusing on sex-drug behavior too early on might prematurely terminate the treatment process.

In working with men and their sexual activity, it is imperative to think of sexualization in the context of sexual orientation (Shelby, 1997). Orientation, "the capacity to fall in love with a person of a particular gender" (Money, 1985) and the defensive use of sexuality are not synonymous. We are attempting to lay out a perspective that does not "privilege" heterosexuality or homosexuality or bisexuality (Chodorow 1992) but enables a focus on the role of the behavior in the maintenance of the self. While different people may have different views as to what constitutes "kinky" or "perverse" or "sexualized" behavior, ultimately, to not explore sexuality in the clinical encounter may be turning away from the patient's distress. For some patients sexuality is the prime vehicle for managing distress. A subset of these patients may require substance use as the most effective coping strategy that they know. The drug use promotes seemingly uninhibited sex, lacking acknowledgement of HIV infection risk, sexual negotiation or condom use. Seemingly, because, how can sex that is propelled by drugs to manage a vulnerable self be truly uninhibited? We must remember that we are encouraging people to be anxious about some forms of sexuality, given the potential for HIV/STD infection. Some people find this "intrusion" intolerable and will attempt to manage its influence by using substances that help them disavow or ignore the dangerous possibilities inherent in their favorite form of sexual activity and associated fantasies.

An intriguing aspect of the research findings by Ostrow and McKirnan was that episodes of unsafe sex and drug use were sporadic rather than consistent. This plus the fact that disinhibiting or dissociative drugs were often employed indicates, from an analytic perspective, that unsafe sex and drug usage may have occurred in the context of an effort to manage distress. A relationship that ends with disappointment and the beginning of a new relationship with all its hope and anxiety are both often destabilizing to the sense of self. Life in general is fraught with frustration, and some people may have difficulty traversing certain developmental phases. Some people will turn to sexuality as a way of managing distressing points in their lives. A patient once referred to his episodes of alcohol and drug use and seeking out a sexual partner as a "sex tantrum." These episodes were in marked contrast to his day-to-day functioning. In retrospect, he thought he had behaved oddly, but when the need to get intoxicated and find a sexual partner emerged, it took on great urgency. Clinical work eventually revealed that he was trying to express a certain sexual fantasy, but also that these episodes occurred during times of stress.

In the clinical encounter, the task becomes not only engaging the patient in reflecting on his behaviors, but to do it in such a way that vulnerable aspects of self may become the point of focus. As we see in the case of Mr. A, his ability to engage the clinician was tenuous, just as his ability to engage other men in sexual encounters was tenuous. He could barely speak to me many times, just as he was afraid to speak to his partners. Despite his outwardly robust appearance, Mr. A was convinced he was a "sissy." On one hand, it was a painful secret; on the other, he was sure that all the world would see it and attack if he were not careful. We often hear of the hope of many traumatized young gay men: that once they move to the big city and immerse themselves in the gay community, they will no longer have to worry about being verbally or physically assaulted for their "difference." However, these old painful feelings often return and color their interactions with other gay men. Considerable anxiety is often present in the bar, circuit party and athletic venues. While we can focus on ageism and competition for the most physically attractive partners as the source of distress, these are external, social explanations. Indeed in the clinical setting, we often encounter men who are physically quite desirable, yet they feel acutely inadequate. Social forces may enhance these vulnerabilities, but we invariably find the roots of these feelings in childhood. Much has been made of the circuit party phenomena where a prime motivation is to merge into a totemic group, dancing as a hypnotic mass, feeling released from a sense of singleness by becoming a part of the huge group. Clinical experience indicates that a good deal of sex and party drugs can be found at athletic events such as softball, volleyball and the rodeos. People bring to these venues their own hopes, fears and vulnerabilities. Alcohol and recreational drugs are often the prime vehicle for managing the distress of coping with so many people, potential alienation, the hope of being accepted, and often the hope of being wanted by another man.

Mr. A used drugs and alcohol to fortify him as he was out and about in the gay community. Instead of the hoped for feelings of acceptance, he was anxious and fearful and fearing rejection. In order for the treatment to proceed, Mr. A first needed to be assured that his therapist could bear and accept these painful, humiliating feelings and not re-traumatize him. With men such as Mr. A, the challenge for the therapist is to act in such a way that the patient does not feel criticized, attacked or rejected, which would repeat in the treatment the very dynamic that played a role in the formation of distressed feelings about the self. Shelby (1999) points out that when the patient is able to talk about their sexualizations, it is often an opportunity to deepen the alliance and transferences, not a call to make the person stop what they are doing. Mr. A needed the therapist to accept his feeling like a sissy: not to do so would be ignoring his distress. However, the therapist also needed to act with him in such a way to not reconfirm his experience of being an incompetent sissy.

Mr. A was quite aware that he was putting himself at risk for contracting HIV, and this was expressed in his anxious somatic complaints as well as the clinical dialogue. Engaging in risky sex enhanced his sense of incompetence as did his frequent episodes of becoming overwhelmed at work. He did not have to be "coached" in how to deal with men, or lectured on safe sex practices. Rather allowing an idealizing transference to unfold at its own pace enabled a gradual strengthening of his self and a gradual decline in episodes of fragmentation or "falling apart." This in turn enabled him to use the knowledge regarding transmission and how to protect himself that he already possessed, and Mr. A came to view talking about safe sex as a sign of competence. Clearly, Mr. A had areas of considerable competence, but these were split off or disavowed and not readily experienced as part of his self. His ability to bring the childhood fantasy of the flying chair into the relationship, signaled a beginning acknowledgment of his own competence and need for his competence to be acknowledged by me. We never know exactly how this will be played out in treatment, but for Mr. A it was planning a long desired trip that he was convinced was beyond his capacity. Confessing to his fluency in French was almost as difficult as relating his difficulties with men.

In summarizing the case, treatment did not focus on the behavioral "symptoms" of alcohol and drug use or placing himself at risk for HIV/STD infection which resulted in distress and somatic fears, but rather the overall vulnerabilities of the self. It approached the motivations to use alcohol and cocaine as he attempted to meet other men. Why he put himself at risk was certainly a central question, but the initial effort was to understand this in the context of his self organization. This is not an encouragement to ignore risky behavior, and we are not opposed to asking a patient, "What is the big deal about using a condom?" when the therapist is attempting to grasp the vulnerabilities that prevent the person from using the knowledge readily available to them. Engaging a fragile and vulnerable person in treatment is often a slow and delicate process. Listening to the emerging transferences rather than focusing on symptoms leads to an encounter that ultimately offers greater access to self structures that are responsible for difficulties engaging others. A silent idealizing transference allows for the stabilization of self states, while a later mirroring transference allows for the expression and integration of his abilities and more stable self esteem. As these occurred, in Mr. A's treatment his need for recreational drugs diminished. Granted, we encounter men who have become addicted to substances, and treatment must first focus on the addiction, often in a program specific to detoxification. However, even in cases of severe addiction, understanding the motivations for the substance use remains a crucial aspect of the treatment. Again, we often observe considerable difficulty in negotiating sexual activity in people after they have relinquished their drug use. Clinical experience indicates that many instances of relapse into drug use occur around attempts to seek out and manage a relationship. Hence, attending to the motivations and needs of the self are integral to any treatment effort. As Mr. A became more comfortable with himself, and consequently less afraid of what others may see, his need to manage his anxiety through drug use declined. While annoying aspects of "reality" may be disavowed in some forms of sexualization, tender feelings and longings are often disavowed as well. Mr. A was ultimately seeking prolonged contact with another man, but felt this too was a sign of weakness. Helping Mr. A acknowledge his longings as part of being human, rather than being a sissy, enabled him to discover that other men were after the same thing as well.

CASE EXAMPLE #2 AND RE-INTRODUCTION OF COGNITIVE-BEHAVIORAL MODELS

Case #2: Mr. F is a single, 35 y/o, Italian-American male who was referred to one of us (DGO) for the treatment of recurrent episodes of alcohol and psychostimulant abuse and for depression. While the depression was related to his recent separation from his wife and her refusal to allow him visitation privileges with their 7 year old son, the drinking/cocaine-amphetamine snorting binges fit a pattern of episodic poly-drug abuse that had begun in his mid-teens and gradually worsened during the past 20 years. There was a strong family history of alcoholism and both the patient and his 3 brothers had worked in the family restaurant business where heavy drinking was the norm. Motivation to treatment was the threat by Mr. F's wife that he would never gain visitation rights if he continued to drink and fear that he would lose his job in the family business as well as his rent-free house and car if he continued to be absent from his job for periods of 5-10 days at a time.

Mr. F denied any episodes of homosexual sex, but his recent drinking/snorting binges had all been precipitated by arguments with his wife and subsequent hooking up with his neighborhood "buddies" who would supply him with alcohol and cocaine until Mr. F ran out of money or blacked out. His cocaine/amphetamine use was secondary to the binge alcohol abuse as the stimulants were used to enable him to continue drinking for 5-10 days at a time without sleeping. In the course of the initial assessment interview, Mr. F also revealed that he had recently been diagnosed as having chronic Hepatitis C (HCV) infection, which he related to the sharing of needles with the same drinking buddies when he took illegal steroids for body building and increased sexual stamina. He estimated that he had had between 150-200 different sexual partners during each of the past 4-5 years, with an estimated total of 2,000 lifetime female sex partners. He did not verbalize any guilt or remorse regarding any of these activities, although his affect was predominantly a mixture of sadness and anger at his wife.

The initial problem list included adjustment disorder with depression; familial binge alcoholism; psychostimulant abuse; steroid abuse; Don Juanism; and chronic HCV infection that could be exacerbated by continued alcoholism. The therapist's initial behavioral concerns included Mr. F's risk of spreading HCV to his many female sexual partners as well as the permanent damage he could cause to both his liver and his role as a father to his son if he continued to drink. Taking a purely cognitive-behavioral approach to treatment would mean that the focus would be on Mr. F's drinking behaviors and the circumstances (anger at wife, desire to be with his male buddies, sadness at being separated from his son) that triggered or facilitated his drinking and snorting binges. However, from an *escape model* perspective it was clear that all of these problem behaviors as well as his promiscuous sexuality could be seen as attempts to escape from the constraints of his marriage and the family business in order to cope with intense feelings of inadequacy that he felt in his roles as father, provider, husband, and, ultimately, as a "whole" man.

From the AIM Model perspective, it is clear that the urgency of Mr. F's pleas for help in halting his rapid downhill slide required immediate supportive psychotherapy and vigorous treatment of both the depression and the urges to drink in order to "drown" his profound depressive symptoms. From a social network and enabler perspective, it was necessary to help Mr. F find alternative networks of friends and companions that would not encourage his drinking/drugging and marathon sexual episodes. Only after Mr. F's situation had been stabilized and his depression/negative self-image treated with combination psychotherapy/antidepressant therapy/group (AA) social support was he able to get in touch with his profound anger and resentment towards his parents for providing him with a lifestyle permissive of and supportive of his drinking, drugging, and sexual exploits. In contrast to the case of Mr. A above, Mr. F presented with specific behavioral intervention needs that required emergency attention and which he could precisely articulate. By helping him to re-organize his life to meet those needs, he could develop a nurturing transference with his therapist and gradually shift the focus of his treatment to the psychodynamic issues which underlie his problematic behaviors. After six months of therapy without any drug abuse, Mr. F was able to taper off his antidepressant treatment but continues in weekly psychotherapy.

DISCUSSION

These two cases were chosen to illustrate the complementary as well as divergent aspects of the cognitive-behavioral and psychoanalytical approaches to the treatment of sex and drug use issues among men. That one of the case studies was a gay male and the other a heterosexual male intentionally illustrates that neither of these issues is an exclusive problem of gay or bisexual men and that while "internalized homophobia" (Shidlo, 1994) may contribute to low self-esteem among gay men, there are other sources of low self-esteem that can apply to heterosexual and homosexual men alike. Additionally, there are many ways people manage self esteem issues. Sexuality and drug use is but one of many possibilities for overcoming distressed affects. And while concern about HIV infection or transmission has motivated many gay or bisexual men to seek treatment for their sex and drug behaviors, concern about HCV infection and/or marital issues can similarly motivate heterosexual or bisexual men.

The AIM Project has revealed much information about the different drugs that gay or bisexual men use to enhance sexual pleasure or to disinhibit their otherwise protective use of condoms (McKirnan et al., 1999). For most straight men, fear of HIV is not a salient enough motivation for them to begin to use condoms consistently, but increasing information in the popular press (e.g., *Details*, *Rolling Stone*, and *Time Magazine* have all recently highlighted HCV among heterosexuals) is beginning to motivate men with multiple partners to seek testing and adopt protective sexual and drug use behaviors. Perhaps, as concern about the seriousness of HIV infection decreases among gay men, leading to reported increases in unprotected anal intercourse and "barebacking," educational campaigns that stress the seriousness of HCV and other sexually transmitted diseases will help to maintain otherwise eroding community norms about the importance of safer sex. Certainly, in our clinical practices, we cannot adopt a complacent attitude towards preventing the widespread return to the sexual and drug use behaviors of the "Pre-AIDS" era. Approaches that strive for understanding the conscious and unconscious motivations for our patients' drug use and sexual behaviors does not mean that we either condone or condemn them.

The fetishizing of barebacking is itself a fascinating phenomenon that needs to be looked at from both the psychoanalytical and cognitive behavioral perspectives. If one examines a barebacking page on the internet, it looks like any other area devoted to fetishes, including stories extolling its virtues, erotic photographs illustrating the activity and personal ads of devotees. However, if one talks to self-identified "barebackers," this writer (DGO) is impressed by their active sense of "revolt" against what they view as "the tyranny of condoms" and long-term dissatisfaction with protected intercourse in casual sexual encounters. For a self-psychology or ego vulnerability understanding of self avowed barebackers, one must consider the inadequacy of HIV/STD prevention programs that rely primarily on fear. These approaches do not address the group identification needs of men whose self-esteem is maintained primarily through their sexuality (Odets, 1994). Such individuals will neither present for individual psychotherapy nor volunteer for group discussions on safer sex issues as for them the issue is not staying HIV negative or not infecting others, but rather, the reassertion of their assumed right to engage in patently unsafe sexual behaviors in the face of opposition by the larger community (Gendlin, 1999; Scarce, 1999). While barebackers may adamantly defend their rights, one does wonder whom they are rebelling against? Is it indeed the emergency safer sex educational efforts that emerged in the 1980s or is it something else?

Clinical work that encounters men who use drugs in the course of their sexual activity is not confined to the consulting room. Community agencies and outreach programs that work with people on their own turf inevitably encounter the complex phenomena of drug use and sexuality. While two very different models have been presented, the ultimate issue is clinical utility. For some men, who are able to openly talk about their sex-drug use behaviors and HIV/STD risk-taking in front of other gay/bisexual men, group therapy formats that focus on teaching them how to safely achieve their intimacy needs are appropriate. For others, who are more fragile and would not be able to tolerate a group format, individual psychotherapy is indicated. Here as well, some people would not be able to tolerate the slow and potentially painful and frustrating process of analytically oriented psychotherapy, and the more focused approach of cognitive behavioral therapy that incorporates self psychological and escape motivation concepts may be more suitable (Ostrow, McKirnan & Hope, 1997). The ultimate issue is not theoretical superiority, rather clinical utility given the population, setting and individual patients. Behavioral research can inform analytic work, just as analytic theory can inform and be used to interpret behavioral research findings.

Sexuality is an important dimension of being human and for many people psychoactive substances are an integral aspect of sexual expression. Whether it is a bottle of Champagne and *Bolero* or crystal methamphetamine and house music, we often observe a linkage between sexuality and a substance that disinhibits, enhances or propels. The problem comes from the ongoing expression of unfettered sexuality in communities with elevated rates of HIV and other infectious agents. The clinician's task then becomes intervening with these populations not as enforcers of the social order, but primarily concerned with alleviating distress by facilitating understanding and new ways of managing distress. We hope that the dialectical examination of actual cases from our clinical practices enhances the ability of practitioners to reduce distress and increase understanding among persons engaging in unsafe sex while under the influence of drugs.

REFERENCES

Center for Substance Abuse Prevention (CSAP), *Alcohol, Tobacco, and other Drugs Resource Guide. Lesbians, Gay Men and Bisexuals.* PHS/USPHHS/SAMHSA Publication No. SMA 94-2097.

Chesney, M., Barrett, D., and Stall, R. (1998), Histories of substance use and risk behavior: Precursors to seroconversion in homosexual men. *American Journal of Public Health*, 88:113-116.

Chodorow, N. (1992), Heterosexuality as a compromise formation: Reflections on the psychoanalytic theory of sexual development. *Psychoanalysis and Contemporary Thought.* 15 (3):267-304.

Dax, E.M., Alder, W.H., Nagel, J.E. et al. (1991), Amyl nitrite alters human in vitro immune function. *Immunopharmacology and Immunotoxicology*, 13:577-587.

Freud, S. (1896), The aetiology of hysteria. *Standard Edition*, 3, 189.

Freud, S. (1905), Three essays on the theory of sexuality. *Standard Edition*, 7, 125.

Freud, S. (1926), Inhibitions, symptoms and anxiety. *Standard Edition*, 20, 77.

Gendlin, S. (1999), They shoot barebackers, don't they? *Poz Magazine*, February, 48-51, 69.

Goldberg, A. (1972), A fresh look at perverse behavior. *International Journal of Psycho-analysis* 56:335-42.

Goldberg, A. (1995), *The problem of perversion.* New Haven, CT: Yale University Press.

May, R. (1995), Re-Reading Freud on homosexuality. In *Disorienting sexuality*, T. Domenici and R. Lesser (eds). New York:Routledge.

McKirnan, D.J., Ostrow, D.G., and Hope, B. (1996), Sex, drugs, and escape: A psychological model of HIV-risky sexual behaviors. *AIDS Care*, 8:655-669.

McKirnan, D.J., Vanable, P.A, Ostrow, D.G., and Hope, B. (1999, submitted), Cognitive escape and sexual risk among drug and alcohol-involved gay and bisexual men.

Money, J. (1988), *Gay, straight, and in-between*. Oxford: Oxford University Press.

Odets, W. (1994), AIDS education and harm reduction for gay men: Psychological approaches for the 21st century. *AIDS & Public Health Policy Journal*, 9:1-18.

Ostrow D.G., Van Raden M.J., Fox R., Kingsley L.A., Dudley J., Kaslow R.A. (1990), Recreational drug use and sexual behavior change in a cohort of homosexual men. *AIDS 4* (8): 759-765.

Ostrow, D.G., DiFranceisco, W., Chmiel, J.S., Wagstaff, D., and Wesch, J. (1995), A case-control study of HIV-1 seroconversion and risk-related behaviors in the Chicago MACS/CCS cohort, 1984-1992. *American J Epidemiology*, 142:875-883.

Ostrow, D.G. (2000), The role of drugs in the sexual lives of MSM: Continuing barriers to researching this question. *AIDS and Behavior*, 4, 205-219.

Ostrow, D.G. and McKirnan, D.J. (1997), Prevention of substance-related high-risk sexual behavior among gay men: Critical review of the literature and proposed harm reduction approach. *Journal of the Gay & Lesbian Medical Association*, 1:97-110.

Scarce, M. (1999), A ride on the wild side: An HIV prevention activist goes through the latex looking glass to discover who's doing it raw, and why. *POZ* (February 1999): 52-55, 70-71.

Shelby, R.D. (1997), The Self and Orientation: The Case of Mr. G. A. Goldberg (ed.) *Progress in Self Psychology*, (12) 55-74.

Shelby, R.D. (1999), *About Cruising and Being Cruised*. Unpublished Manuscript.

Shidlo, A. (1994), Internalized homophobia. Conceptual and empirical issues in measurement. In B. Greene and G.M. Herek (Eds.). *Lesbian and Gay Psychology. Theory, Research, and Clinical Applications*. Thousand Oaks, CA; Sage Publications; pp. 176-205.

Stall, R., McKusick, L., Wiley, J., Coates, T.J., and Ostrow, D.G. (1986), Alcohol and drug use during sexual activity and compliance with safe sex guidelines for AIDS: The AIDS Behavioral Research Project. *Health Education Quarterly*, 13:359-372.

Stall, R., and Purcell, D. (2000), Intertwining epidemics: A review of research on substance use among men who have sex with men and its connection to the AIDS epidemic. *AIDS and Behavior*.

Stoller, R. (1975), *Perversion: The erotic form of hatred*. New York: Pantheon.

Tolpin, M. (1997), Sexuality and the self. *Annual of Psychoanalysis*, 15:173.

Watson. R.R. (1990, Ed.), *Cofactors in HIV Infection and AIDS*. Boca Raton, FL, CRC Press.

Sexual Compulsivity in Gay Men from a Jungian Perspective

John A. Gosling, MD

SUMMARY. This paper offers an approach to the understanding and psychotherapeutic treatment from a Jungian perspective of gay men who seek treatment for sexual compulsivity. It presents a definition of sexual compulsivity that places it in the diagnostic category of an addiction. A classification from an affect theory perspective is presented to clarify the different variants of sexual compulsivity. The paper focuses primarily on two specific types of sexual compulsivity: (1) Sexual encounters for the purpose of avoiding discomforting "unacceptable" repressed affects. This is the result of the psychological mechanism of splitting and repression that causes sexual energy and other vital affects to be repressed in the unconscious where they constellate as part of the shadow. This repressed shadow aspect, driven by sexual energy, takes on a negative form in the unconscious and can at times function independently of the ego resulting in loss of control and sexual compulsivity. (2) Sexual encounters driven by an addiction to the affect of excitement. Unconscious archetypal masculine energy is projected onto the phallus of any anonymous sex partner where it is "worshipped" and experienced as charged with numinous energy. Because of the lack of awareness of and the paucity of outlets for the experience of the numinous in our desacrelized society, being in the presence of this powerful numinous energy is extremely compelling and exciting and paves the way for sexual compulsivity. As awareness of wounding of the archetypal masculine energy is recognized in the course of therapy, the possibility for this energy's positive attributes to

---

Dr. John A. Gosling is a Psychiatrist/Jungian Analyst in New York, NY.

[Haworth co-indexing entry note]: "Sexual Compulsivity in Gay Men from a Jungian Perspective." Gosling, John A. Co-published simultaneously in *Journal of Gay & Lesbian Psychotherapy* (The Haworth Medical Press, an imprint of The Haworth Press, Inc.) Vol. 3, No. 3/4, 2000, pp. 141-167; and: *Addictions in the Gay and Lesbian Community* (ed: Jeffrey R. Guss, and Jack Drescher) The Haworth Medical Press, an imprint of The Haworth Press, Inc., 2000, pp. 141-167. Single or multiple copies of this article are available from The Haworth Document Delivery Service [1-800-342-9678, 9:00 a.m. - 5:00 p.m. (EST). E-mail address: getinfo@haworthpressinc.com].

© 2000 by The Haworth Press, Inc. All rights reserved.

141

emerge in the life experience of the individual becomes a reality. He is able to reclaim his own power and this helps improve self-esteem.

Jung's concept of a teleological or synthetic approach to treatment (including the use of active imagination) is explored and illustrated in a clinical case study. His concept of the numinous and how it possibly relates to sexual compulsivity is discussed. Shame as an important etiological factor is emphasized. The concept of the shadow, including its necessary integration in the course of treatment, is discussed. The epic of *Gilgamesh* is used as a helpful tool in the treatment process of the clinical case presented. Following the bibliography, an appendix has been added. This is a response from the person who was discussed in the clinical case after he read the paper and also includes comments on his impressions of the treatment process. *[Article copies available for a fee from The Haworth Document Delivery Service: 1-800-342-9678. E-mail address: <getinfo@haworthpressinc.com> Website: <http://www.HaworthPress.com>]*

KEYWORDS. Sexual compulsivity, gay men, Jung, acting out, psychotherapy, dreams, and homosexuality

The discussion will follow the following format: (1) Definition of sexual compulsivity; (2) Classification from the perspective of affect theory; (3) Discussion of Jung's concept of a teleological approach to treatment; (4) Shame as a contributing etiological factor; (5) The epic of *Gilgamesh*; (6) A clinical case study: Paul; (7) Conclusion; (8) Bibliography; and (9) Appendix: Response from Paul.

DEFINITION

Sexual compulsivity is often diagnosed as a form of impulse disregulation that results in compulsive sexual acting out behavior that the person feels driven to perform and over which he feels he has little or no control. If this causes the person distress, it can be diagnosed according to the criteria in the DSM-IV, as Sexual Disorder Not Otherwise Specified. However, the essential features of all substance-use disorders according to the DSM-IV are the following: (1) loss of control, (2) preoccupation with, and (3) repetition of the behavior in spite of adverse consequences. These criteria apply to many cases of sexually compulsive behavior as well so that it can thus also be regarded as an addictive disorder.

CLASSIFICATION FROM AN AFFECT THEORY PERSPECTIVE

From an affect theory perspective four types of affect dynamics are described (Kaufman and Raphael, 1996, 214-221), which provide a helpful framework within which to contextualize sexual addiction:

Sex as a Sedative

Most addictions rely on a particular sedative–alcohol, drugs, food, cigarettes, shopping, or sex–to reduce or suppress being overwhelmed and discomforted by certain affects. These disturbing affects may be shame, rage, fear, loneliness, sadness or any other intolerable affects. In some cases the sedative effect of some form of sexual activity may have initially been used for comfort in the presence of negative affect situations, such as humiliating shame, ridicule, rejection, or hurt. Sexual activity may have been used initially to comfort wounds caused by significant losses, such as the death of a beloved parent, sibling or loved one. Compulsive sexual activity could also mask the symptoms of an undiagnosed clinical depression. Sex may be used in the service of self-medicating and bring about temporary relief of the discomforting affects associated with depression.

If used repeatedly for this purpose of avoidance of discomforting affects, the sexual activity that was initially experienced as soothing and comforting becomes a behavior that appears to ward off negative or intolerable affects. Eventually, the absence of the sedative effect of sex causes increasing anxiety that can only be relieved by more sex. Sexual addiction has set in when the person learns that being deprived of the sedative effect of sex is much worse than any other negative affects that it may reduce (Kaufman and Raphael, 1996, 217). The addiction to the sedative effect of sex becomes so powerful that it overrides rationality. The person may then engage in potentially dangerous and self-destructive behaviors such as exposure to HIV or to other potentially dangerous situations. He may also risk disruption or loss of his relationship with a primary partner. The addictive behavior becomes an all-consuming activity over which he feels he has little or no control.

Harry described his experience as follows:

> When I was about five years old, my parents caught me with another little boy under the bed with our pants down. They forced me to walk around naked in the house as punishment. I remember feeling so ashamed. To comfort myself I masturbated that day as soon as I could. After this I began masturbating all the time, several times per day. It made me feel better. It was a comfort to me. I still find myself doing this now when I am upset.

For Harry, masturbation initially was a way of comforting himself as a child in a situation that caused extreme negative affect, namely, shame and humiliation. He subsequently found it to be a source of comfort throughout his childhood. In adolescence and adulthood, sex continued to bring about immediate, though temporary, relief from feeling "upset." It had a sedative effect and helped suppress intolerable or unpleasant affects. As an adult, he gradually began to notice that when unable to have sex he felt increasingly anxious. The absence of the sedative and comforting effect of sex now produced intense discomfort, a critical factor in the shift from sedation to addiction (Kaufman and Raphael, 1996, 216). This could only be relieved by more sex. Harry had become addicted to sex.

In childhood and adolescence, the expression of any affect or instinctual energy (such as sexuality) that is met with ridicule or other negative reaction often results in the psychological mechanism of dissociation and repression. Such dissociative splits with repression of affects and instinctual energy, results in an inability to access or express these powerful energies appropriately. However, without access to the entire spectrum of affects and instinctual energies, the capacity for intimacy, relatedness and love is significantly jeopardized. The repressed affects constellate in the unconscious giving rise to problematic complexes that often exert a powerful negative influence on the conscious ego, giving rise to acting out behaviors over which the person feels he has limited control. The split off sexual energy often tends to take on a life of its own and results in sexual acting out and/or compulsivity. (This is discussed below in reference to the shadow.)

This dissociative split with subsequent repression occurs in many persons but particularly in gay men when the expression of sexual energy that is homoerotic is shamed into the unconscious. Often a vicious cycle is set in motion: the expression of sexual feelings, having previously been met with shame and/or ridicule give rise to overwhelming feelings of shame; sexual activity provides comfort for this discomforting affect–which in turn elicits further shame that is relieved by more sex. A pattern of repetition compulsion takes hold and sexual addiction follows. As the capacity to tolerate bringing repressed affects and sexual energies into awareness develops in the course of therapy and recovery, there is increasingly less need to engage in sedative sexual addictive behaviors. The ability to express a full range of affects more appropriately and the capacity to embrace the expression of sexuality without shame can allow the person to be more fully related. Intimacy in relationships becomes possible and sexuality no longer needs to be split off and lead an independent life of its own. Establishing and maintaining loving relationships that include the freedom to express affects and sexuality becomes a possibility.

Sex Used to Release Suppressed Affect

Sexual activity (and other addictive behaviors) can also be used for the release of affect that has had to be chronically suppressed. Sex then serves the purpose of being a dis-inhibitor of suppressed affect. This is a well-recognized effect of the use of alcohol, although the biochemical pathways and mechanism of action by which alcohol brings about its disinhibition is quite different from that of sex. A sexual encounter can provide a forum where a person with overly suppressed affects can allow themselves to actually express affects of various kinds. If sex becomes associated with the release of suppressed affect and is perceived as the only available means to do this, the person can become addicted to sex in order to be able to express feelings that cannot find an outlet elsewhere (Kaufman and Raphael, 1996, 218).

Adam grew up in an abusive household. His father physically and emotionally abused him. His mother failed to protect him and would also beat him. His beloved grandmother however, adored him. She treated him like a little prince. He came to understand that an important aspect of his sexual addiction was related to experiencing affects that he otherwise was unable to feel. In the course of a sexual encounter he felt affirmed, attractive and adored. These were the positive affects that he had felt when with his grandmother. When not engaged in sex, he suffered from low self-esteem, was hypercritical of himself and felt much guilt and shame. Sex was the only place where he could connect with the suppressed positive affects associated with his grandmother. He came to need sex to boost his self-esteem. Adam was not using sex to sedate his feelings but to experience suppressed affects that he otherwise could not access.

Sex and the Affect of Excitement

Another type of affect dynamic that may be operating in sexual addictions is addiction to the affect of excitement experienced in the sexual encounter. In order to sustain the excitement affect, many and varied sexual partners are required to maintain the passionate thrill of sex with a stranger. This gives rise to indiscriminate promiscuity. There is a hunger for ever-increasing levels of excitement that can only be experienced with new sexual partners. This form of sexual addictive behavior will be expanded upon below. I am postulating the hypothesis that the numinous inner image of archetypal masculine energy (*Phallos*) in the unconscious is projected onto the phallus (the erect penis) of the sex partner where it is "worshipped." The person is usually totally unaware of this unconscious dynamic. Consciously they would only be seeking a sexual encounter. The excitement affect that results in these situations is in part the result of being in the presence of powerful numinous energy (see below) which has a transpersonal quality to it. Connecting with this energy is highly addictive because of the hunger in our desacrelized society for a connection with spiritual or transpersonal energies. As mentioned above, this form of addiction results in promiscuity because only sex with a stranger can sustain the dynamic of projection accompanied by an experience of the numinous. Once familiarity takes place, the projection of numinous archetypal masculine energy onto the phallus of the sex partner is more difficult to sustain and hence the excitement affect diminishes. Because one of the features of persons who have symptoms of Attention-Deficit Disorder (ADD) is the craving for excitement from risk-taking behaviors, they may be more vulnerable to this form of sexual addiction.

Kaufman and Raphael (1996, 219) point out that the quest for excitement can totally dominate a person's life. All other affects are subjugated to the thrill of anonymous sex. It can even endanger the enjoyment of relatedness in more enduring relationships. In this type of addiction, sex is neither a sedative nor a dis-inhibitor of suppressed affect, but instead becomes an all-consuming uncontrollable quest for greater experiences of excitement.

One of the challenges in recovering from this form of sexual addiction is the process of learning to become less addicted to the experience of excitement affect in anonymous sexual encounters. The person begins to be able to cultivate the awareness of other affects, such as enjoyment and pleasure in the context of more enduring relationships. It becomes possible to also have numinous experiences that are not only sexual in nature. As the person is able to recognize the projection of his own positive inner masculine energies onto the phallus of strangers, the possibility of expressing these attributes in himself leads to empowerment and improved self-esteem. He is able to be more accepting of who he is (including his sexual orientation). The experience of being "out" and taking a stand for his beliefs in the face of possible adversity becomes a reality. Creativity is more accessible and there is a willingness to bring this forth and for it to be seen in the world. There is an increased ability to be aware of his needs and to express them appropriately. He is also better able to protect himself from abuse and re-wounding, especially in the area of his sexuality. He may finally be able to experience a sense of pride in his achievements: "Here I stand. I can be no other." This reduces the need to concretize and literalize these intrapsychic functions by projecting these qualities onto the phallus of a stranger. There is a concomitant reduction in shame and the possibility of making more conscious choices becomes an option.

Twelve Step programs, such as Sexual Compulsives Anonymous (S.C.A.), or Sexual Addicts Anonymous (S.A.A.), that encourage the awareness of spiritual or transpersonal energies may be particularly helpful in supporting recovery from this type of sexual addiction. These programs acknowledge "that a Power greater than ourselves could restore us to sanity." Members are encouraged to seek "through prayer and meditation to improve our conscious contact with God, *as we understand God.*" Part of the recovery process is thus a more conscious acknowledgement of and connection with whatever God or Higher Power may represent to each person. This may be a more conscious relationship with the authentic inner self (the Self or archetype of wholeness described by Jung) and other powerful forces in the unconscious; an awareness of spirituality and transpersonal connections in everyday life and in nature; or the expression of creativity. Specific workshops are offered by SCA on ways to connect with the numinous energy of Higher Power other than through anonymous sexual encounters. Some gay men in recovery from sexual compulsivity have found these workshops to be very beneficial.

Sex and the Displacement of Affect

The last type of affect management that may give rise to sexual addiction is the displacement of suppressed affect into sex and its expression via sexual activity. If one is criticized or humiliated in some situation where the resulting discomforting affect of shame cannot be expressed (in the work situation, for example) and is suppressed, a degrading sexual encounter may serve to discharge this affect (Kaufman and Raphael, 1996, 220). The sexual humiliation results in an intensification of the shame. Shame is displaced into the sex and expressed in this context rather than in the original situation. Addiction to this type of sexual encounter may ensue if it becomes the only outlet for certain intense affects such as shame and humiliation that cannot be expressed in other ways. This dynamic may give rise to various forms of sadomasochistic patterns. The painful affect of shame becomes eroticized in an encounter where the person is sexually humiliated. Alternatively, one person may identify with the aggressor and assume the dominant powerful role and humiliate the other person sexually.

In this article, I will focus mainly on the first and third forms of sexual addiction according to the above classification, namely, sexual encounters used in the service of avoiding discomforting affects and the addiction to the affect of excitement. Although the above classification according to affect theory provides a useful framework outlining various mechanisms involved in sexual addiction, most persons seeking treatment do not fit into any single category. The human psyche is extremely complex and each person presents their own unique multiplicity of determining factors and modes of expression.

A TELEOLOGICAL APPROACH TO TREATMENT

It is always important to attempt to make a definitive diagnosis when treating someone for sexual compulsivity. The above definition and affect dynamics serve as helpful guidelines in understanding variations in the various presentations of sexual compulsivity compelling someone to seek treatment. The approach to treatment will largely be determined by the theoretical orientation of the therapist. Jung used the word "reductive" to describe the process of attempting to reveal the primitive, instinctual, infantile or other possible childhood experiences as the causes of the person's current symptoms. Jung was critical of using only the reductive method because he contended that it did not explore the full meaning of the symptom or behavior.

He was more interested in exploring where the person's life was leading them than focussing on the causes of how they had arrived at that point. His was a teleological point of view. Jung described this orientation as "synthetic" with the implication that what emerged from the starting point of treatment was of primary significance and moved the process forward. His interest was mainly in the unique constellation of the intrapsychic energies in a particular individual at the time that they presented for treatment. Viewed from this unique perspective that is teleological rather than purely reductive, an attempt is made to understand the symptoms as if they had intention and purpose.

Jung also developed methods for engaging the energies in the unconscious by personifying them as they appeared in dream images as well as in the process of "active imagination." He described this process of active imagination as follows: the person focuses on a specific dream image, mood or event and then allows a dialogue to occur or a chain of associated fantasies (1963, par. 706). The conscious ego is actively engaged in the process and can react more immediately and directly than is the case with dreams. Active imagination can facilitate the process of psychotherapy but it achieves success only if it is integrated and does not become either a substitute for or an escape from the labor of conscious living (Samuels, 1986, 9). This helps the person become more familiar with his inner world and the unconscious forces that profoundly affect behavior. By becoming more familiar with the forces in their unconscious, Jung hoped that the person would form an ongoing relationship with their inner world. This would allow for the possibility of making more conscious choices instead of being at the mercy of unconscious forces over which the person felt they had little or no control. There was also the hope that some of the negative potentially destructive aspects could be transformed into more supportive and positive energies.

From the teleological perspective, Jung tended to place less emphasis on the contribution of traumatic childhood and other experiences or the relationship with the parents. With sexual compulsivity, however, the causes are multiple and complex. The contribution of shaming parents and others in the boy's childhood, toxic homophobia, abuse (emotional, physical or sexual), inherent disposition, and many other factors can all play a role. In the course of my psychotherapeutic work I use an integrative approach of both the reductive method as well as the synthetic or teleological approach, as will become evident from the case material presented below.

Using a teleological approach, sexual compulsivity in some persons may be understood as a powerful urge to connect with "something" that is compelling and fascinating, over which the individual feels he has little or no control. In this context, the basic instinct is sexual in nature and for gay men the compelling object is the phallus. Being in the presence of the phallus can be a "numinous" experience (resulting in a connection with transpersonal or spiritual energies, see below) although the person may not be aware of it. This arouses the affect of excitement. If this is the only way in which the person experiences spiritual or transpersonal energy, the thrill that this causes gives rise to a craving to repeat the experience. The desire for the numinous connection and concomitant arousal may lead to sexual compulsivity. The "symptom" of sexual compulsivity is thus not only to be regarded as the emanation of an underlying disturbance or imbalance, but also as a yearning for an encounter with powerful spiritual or transpersonal energies, in this instance experienced in the presence of an erect phallus. Instead of attaching to religious icons and symbols, this energy becomes attached to the phallus.

Because of the dissociation and repression of sexual energy from consciousness, it tends to function autonomously outside the realm of awareness (the mechanism is discussed below). This is one of the reasons that it can subsume the conscious personality or ego and lead to compulsive behaviors. The repetitive and compulsive nature of this activity can be viewed from a teleological perspective also as an attempt at self-healing. These behaviors may be the result of repeated attempts to comfort the self in the face of discomforting affects, to experience feelings that otherwise cannot be accessed, or to discharge displaced affects (as described above). Because of the loss of conscious control, however, it may also draw the person's attention to the fact that he is out of balance and is suffering from a state of dis-ease and hence may need to seek some form of treatment.

THE NUMINOUS

Jung described the *numinosum* as "either a quality belonging to a visible object or the influence of an invisible presence that causes a peculiar alteration of consciousness" (1958, par. 6). Jung borrowed the word "numinous" from Rudolf Otto's (1926) book *The Idea of the Holy*, which had a major influence on Jung's thought (1950, par. 580, 583; 1958, par. 6, 7, 9, 222 and 472). According to Otto, the essence of holiness, or religious experience, has a specific quality that remains inexpressible and eludes description. To convey its uniqueness, he coined the term "numinous" from the Latin *numen*, meaning a god, cognate with the verb *nuere*, to nod or beckon, indicating divine approval. The numinous is compelling and mysterious. It has the power to attract and to fascinate us. It is alluring. It is non-rational and irreducible. It can only be evoked and experienced (Otto, R, 1926, 7). Once experienced, a longing for it is awakened. It grips the person with a powerful affective state. It allows for a spiritual or transpersonal experience. Otto describes it as follows:

> The feeling of it may at times come sweeping like a gentle tide, pervading the mind with a tranquil mood of deepest worship. It may pass over

into a more set and lasting attitude of the soul, continuing as it were, thrillingly vibrant and resonant, until at last it dies away and the soul resumes its "profane," non-religious mood of everyday experience. *It may burst in sudden eruption up from the depths of the soul with spasms and convulsions, or lead to the strangest excitements, to intoxicated frenzy, to transport, and to ecstasy* (emphasis mine). It has its wild and demonic forms and can sink to an almost grisly horror and shuddering. It has its crude barbaric antecedents and early manifestations, and again it may be developed into something beautiful and pure and glorious. It may become the hushed, trembling and speechless humility of the creature in the presence of–whom or what? In the presence of that which is a *mystery* inexpressible and above all creatures. (1926, 12)

In my opinion, some sexual encounters allow one to satisfy the basic human desire for a numinous experience, to be in the presence of a "mystery inexpressible," that arouses tremendous excitement affect. For some gay men, this numinous experience occurs in the presence of the phallus or erect penis. Others may experience it in the presence of other admired masculine attributes such as a firm muscular torso. The symbol of the phallus in particular is "a pictorial representation of the essence of manliness, a representation of the synthesis of every imaginable aspect of proper manhood" (Vanggaard, 1972, 56). It symbolizes the inner image of archetypal masculinity (*Phallos*) carried in the psyche of every male. In its positive aspects, it represents the willingness to be seen, proudly and assertively; the ability to expose oneself in taking a stand for one's beliefs; the courage to put out into the world one's creative endeavors, and the strength to take responsibility for one's actions.

The phallus has been regarded as a sacred symbol since ancient times. "The phallus is the source of life and libido, the creator and worker of miracles, and as such it was worshipped everywhere" (Jung, 1956, par 146). In Hinduism, the great god Shiva is worshipped in the form of a phallus. Many homes in India have on their shrines a *lingam*, a phallic object, representing the god Shiva. Phallic objects represented the Greek god Dionysus, god of fertility, creativity and ecstasy. A phallus was crowned with wreaths and carried around in the god's cult. During Dionysiac celebrations a song was sung to phallus. There is inscriptional evidence for the use of a large wooden phallus in the processions of the Dionysia in Delos (Otto, W. 164).

As an illustration of how the numinous manifests in our daily lives, some gay men will be able to identify times when overpowering sexual energy has "burst in sudden eruption up from the depths of the soul with spasms and convulsions" (see above quote regarding the numinous). This may lead to "the strangest excitements, to intoxicated frenzy, to transport, and ecstasy." Contemporary humanistic psychology refers to such impressive occurrences as "peak experiences." Eliade, noted historian of religion, states that "except in the modern world, sexuality has everywhere and always been a hierophany (a manifestation of the holy), and the sexual act an integral action and therefore also a means of knowledge" (1969, 14). The spontaneously shared experiences of Joe and Alan that follow serve to further illustrate the manifestation of numinous energy in the daily lives of these two gay men.

Joe was in treatment with me for his sexual addiction. During the course of our work together, he reported the following:

> When I walk down the street, my eyes are always drawn to the crotch of cute boys like magnets. It seems to happen almost automatically. If the guy has a large crotch, I'm immediately entranced. Sometimes I feel compelled to turn around and follow him even if I don't really have the time. It is as though I go into some sort of trance. I am gripped by a feeling of awe that feels out of my control. I want him! I want to worship him!

Alan, who had also sought treatment with me for his sexual addiction, described his experience of a visit to a sex club for gay men, which he frequented on a regular basis. He expressed concern that he was spending too much time there and that it had become part of his sexual addiction. These clubs may be regarded as "temples" where the phallus is worshipped by gay men, albeit unconsciously. They are usually dark and often underground. This phenomenon is indicative of the realm to which sexuality has had to be banished in many gay men, namely, to the darker less conscious regions of the psyche. Alan's description of his experience follows:

> When I'm in the presence of an erect dick (phallus), something happens to me that I find difficult to explain. I start to tremble, quite involuntarily. It's as though I'm in the presence of something greater than me and my little world. I have this indescribable urge to fall to my knees and worship this magnificent object. All the while, I've lost touch with my surroundings. I no longer hear the music. I'm totally unaware of any onlookers. I lose all sense of time. I am taken over by desire, a sort of adoration. I won't bore you with the details of what I want to do with it. I'm in a state of ecstasy (even though I haven't taken any!). It's almost like a religious experience.

In some gay men, numinously charged sexual energy is shamed into the unconscious in childhood or adolescence (as discussed below). I am postulating that this repressed sexual energy constellates in the unconscious around the archetype of the inner phallic god-image (*Phallos*) present in the psyche of every male (Monick, 1987, 16) and becomes part of what Jung calls the shadow. Jung explains this phenomenon of repression of numinous energy as follows:

Since energy never vanishes, the emotional energy that manifests itself in all numinous phenomena does not cease to exist when it disappears from consciousness. As I have said, it reappears in conscious manifestations, in symbolic happenings that compensate the disturbances of the conscious psyche. (1950, par. 583)

The phallus of a stranger and the numinous experience that an encounter with it engenders, becomes the compensatory conscious manifestation of this process. The inner phallic image is projected onto the phallus of strangers where it is "worshipped."

SHAME AS A CONTRIBUTING ETIOLOGICAL FACTOR

A core of shame is often at the root of sexual compulsivity. Gay boys are often confronted at an early age by culturally defined, potentially destructive homophobic or heterosexist attitudes in their parents, family and peers. Being shamed, ridiculed, criticized or even beaten for any gender non-conforming behavior is a frequent occurrence in the lives of gay men. Any expression of perceived homoerotic or "girlish/sissy" behavior often evokes a shaming response. These repeated humiliations result in dissociation and repression of this sexual energy. With repeated shaming (which in many sex addicts is accompanied by a history of sexual and/or physical abuse) the dissociative split and subsequent repression is severe. This defensive survival mechanism serves the purpose of warding off intolerable anxiety associated with these now unacceptable aspects of the self. Using the concept of left (rational, logical, ego, conscious) and right (irrational, instinctual, affective, unconscious) brain hemisphere functions, repeated shaming "damages" and "shuts down" the bridge necessary for communication between these two sides of the brain. Winnicott (1960) describes this defensive split as resulting in the development of a false self with the need to hide the true or authentic self. The sexual energy, primarily governed by the right brain, is separated from the rest of the personality and tends to lead an independent life of its own. The homoerotic/homosexual impulses, which form a vital part of the true self in gay boys, are repressed and go "underground," where they disappear in the deeper layers of the unconscious with unpredictable results.

Having been banished into the nether regions of the unconscious and denied the chance to be expressed in consciousness in an uninhibited fashion, the homoerotic/homosexual energy constellates as an ever present destructive "shadow," primarily in the right brain. Jung points out that even tendencies that might exert a beneficial influence turn into veritable demons when they are repressed (1950, par. 580). Jung's clearest definition of the shadow is as follows: "the thing a person has no wish to be" (1954, par. 470). It is that which one perceives to be one's dark side, the unpleasant or unacceptable qualities one wants to hide. It tends to take on a life of its own, operating from the unconscious, thwarting our most well meant intentions. Given that these particular shadow aspects are sexual in nature, they also become powerfully affectively charged. The shadow tends to function autonomously and is therefore capable of startling and overwhelming the well-ordered ego (Samuels, 1986, 101). When these repressed shadow aspects surface in later life in the form of compulsive sexual acting out behaviors, it leaves the ego feeling helpless and powerless.

To help someone deal with their shadow, it is necessary for the therapist to find a way in which the conscious personality and the shadow can live together (Jung, 1958, par. 132). To become aware of the shadow, to admit to its existence and to attempt a more conscious integration of it is helpful in breaking its compulsive hold. Using the concept of left and right brain hemisphere functions mentioned above, the damage done to the "bridge" between the left brain and the right brain as a result of repeated shaming, resulting in this split, has to be repaired. This occurs in the course of treatment as the person becomes aware of the core of toxic shame and it begins to gradually lessen. The more conscious rational aspect of the ego is repeatedly encouraged to observe and monitor what occurs in the right brain. Input from both sides of the brain is imperative for the mature functioning of the personality. Irrational instincts and powerful affects aroused in the right brain need to be appropriately monitored and managed by the left brain. In order for this to happen, energy needs to be able to flow freely between right and left brain hemispheres across an intact, repaired "bridge." Much of the work in therapy entails a slow and systematic "repair" of this "bridge" so that the split between left brain and right brain functions gradually decreases resulting in a more integrated functional personality. I often find it helpful to use the metaphor of the need to develop an eagle's eye viewpoint, or overview, in order to monitor the "traffic" on the "bridge." This is also referred to as the development of an "observing ego" that is helpful in monitoring and regulating the flow of energy back and forth between left and right brain hemispheres.

Conscious integration of the sexual aspects of the shadow is an important part of the coming out process for gay men. The sexual aspects of the shadow also constitute a vital part of the true or authentic self. It may take many years, perhaps even a lifetime, for the authentic self with its homoerotic and sexual shadow aspects to re-emerge and be reintegrated into the personality. In the therapeutic setting, enormous patience on the part of the therapist is often required to allow the traumatized true self to re-emerge (Drescher, 1998a). The stages of "coming out" and reconnecting with the authentic self is a process and not a one-time event (Drescher 1998a, Scasta, 1998). The same is true of the attempts to become aware of and to integrate the shadow.

By bringing awareness to these "forbidden" desires and repressed affects, the person is better able to make conscious choices.

In order to illustrate this process of integration of the shadow with a clinical example, I will first relate the ancient epic of *Gilgamesh* (Mason, 1970). In my experience, engaging the unconscious by using imagery (the primary language of the unconscious) as portrayed in myths, epics, fairy tales and dreams is a potent clinical tool.

THE EPIC OF GILGAMESH

Myths and epics originated millennia ago as a result of our ancestors' attempts to explain some phenomenon of nature, the origin of humankind, the customs, institutions, or religious rites of a people. Myths and epics usually involve the exploits of gods and heroes, ostensibly with a historical basis. They appear to have evolved as an attempt to explain the peculiarities of observed human behavior using vivid and colorful imagery while at the same time proposing possible solutions to some of life's most difficult challenges such as death, loss and the meaning of life.

The epic of *Gilgamesh* is Sumerian in origin, and is believed to have been created as far back as the third millenium BC (Mason, 98). It predates the Bible and the Homeric epics, the latter by at least a millenium and a half (Mason, 99). It is therefore one of humankind's oldest and most enduring stories. It was later added to and unified as a national epic by the Semitic Babylonians. A number of clay tablets on which the *Gilgamesh* was written were discovered in the nineteenth century in the temple library and palace ruins of Ninevah.

The epic of *Gilgamesh* is divided into several parts and has different subplots. The first section describes the meeting and friendship that develops between Enkidu and Gilgamesh. The friends become inseparable and go on an adventure to slay a troublesome beast, the Evil One named Humbaba, in the forest. Enkidu succeeds in slaying Humbaba and the Bull of Heaven who was sent by the enraged goddess Ishtar after Gilgamesh rejected her advances. During the battles with these beasts, Enkidu is mortally wounded and eventually dies. Gilgamesh is stricken with grief at the death of his friend and is unable to recover from this bitter loss. The rest of the epic is about Gilgamesh's quest to find a way to bring his friend back to life. After many adventures, he succeeds in extracting the knowledge from an old man who tells him that there is a plant in the river that will give him new life. Gilgamesh finds it but leaves it on the side of a stream while he bathes. A serpent smells the plant and devours it. Gilgamesh finds only its shed skin where the plant was. He accepts his fate and limitations and returns to Uruk to rule as king. He has acquired wisdom and the knowledge of the possibility of renewal and rebirth (symbolized by the shed skin of the snake) in the face of loss and grief.

The first part of this epic, namely, the description of Gilgamesh and Enkidu and their meeting and developing friendship, is relevant to illustrate the clinical process of the integration of the shadow mentioned above. The initial separation of Gilgamesh and Enkidu is useful as a metaphor for the dissociative split that occurs in gay men when instinctual sexual energy and other affects are forced into the unconscious (right brain) as a result of shaming or other situations charged with negative affect (as described above). Gilgamesh, king of Uruk, represents the more rational intellectual aspect, or left brain functions, that rules the personality disconnected from sexuality and "unacceptable" affects, or right brain functions. As a result of this split, Gilgamesh is initially described as "a tyrant to his people" (Mason, 15). He "was a godlike man alone with his thoughts in idleness" (Mason, 16-17). He appears to lack a feeling connection to his people and is quite unrelated. Enkidu represents the uninhibited, chthonic, instinctual aspect of the personality that includes the sexual energy and the affects split off from the intellect or more rational aspect of the psyche. "He ran with the animals, drank at their springs, not knowing fear or wisdom" (Mason, 16). This process of dissociative splitting and repression of sexual instinctual energy and other affects can impede linkages between the need for intimacy and sexual feelings (Drescher, 1998b, 286). When disconnected from the instinctual self and the affects, it is difficult to be related to either oneself or to others in a meaningful way. When this split has occurred, these two aspects of the personality tend to operate independently. The "bridge" between left and right brain hemispheres is all but shut down for business, metaphorically speaking. If this split is severe enough, sexual energy (right brain) will tend to usurp the more rational (left brain) part of the personality at times, "not knowing fear or wisdom." Sexual acting out can then occur that is beyond the control of the more conscious rational self. This gives rise to the phenomenon of sexual compulsivity. One of the goals of treatment is to bridge this split between intellect (left brain) and instinct (right brain), the conscious more rational self and the unconscious more instinctual self, resulting in a better integration of the personality. In terms of the epic of *Gilgamesh*, this process is symbolized by the meeting of Gilgamesh and Enkidu and the friendship that develops between them: "It is the story of their becoming human together" (Mason, 15). Their initial encounter is described as follows:

> Gilgamesh looked at the stranger
> And listened to his people's shouts of praise
> For someone other than himself
> And lunged at Enkidu.
> They fell like wolves

At each other's throats,
Like bulls bellowing,
And horses gasping for breath
That have run all day
Desperate for rest and water,
Crushing the gate they fell against.
The dry dust billowed in the marketplace
And people shrieked. The dogs raced
In and out between their legs.
A child screamed at their feet
That danced the dance of life
Which hovers close to death.
And quiet suddenly fell on them
When Gilgamesh stood still
Exhausted. He turned to Enkidu who leaned
Against his shoulder and looked into his eyes
And saw himself in the other, just as Enkidu saw
Himself in Gilgamesh.
In the silence of the people they began to laugh
And clutched each other in their breathless exaltation. (Mason, 23-24)

As will be illustrated in the clinical material presented below, the encounter with the shadow aspect of the personality in personified form is often a frightening experience. The process usually involves repeated confrontations and a considerable struggle until a more conscious integration occurs so that these two aspects of the self can learn to "clutch each other in their breathless exultation."

CLINICAL CASE DISCUSSION: PAUL

Paul sought treatment with me because he was concerned about his sexual compulsivity. He had been attending SCA regularly for several years but in spite of this, he found himself still acting out sexually on occasion. He was in a stable long-term relationship with a partner for several years and was afraid that his sexual compulsivity would ultimately jeopardize his relationship. He suspected that he might be suffering from Attention-Deficit Disorder (ADD) and part of the initial assessment included confirming this diagnosis. He recognized that the impulse disregulation aspect of ADD contributed to his sexually compulsive behavior. He reported that it seemed like there was a separate part of him that would "take over" at times and he'd go into a trance-like state. At these times he was more prone to acting out sexually. Drescher describes this phenomenon as follows:

Some people may experience their sexual desires as a compulsive force, outside their conscious control. Their sexual activities can take place *in a reverie state, a severe dissociative phenomenon that significantly interferes with developing a sense of self.* (emphasis mine) (1998b, 283)

One of Paul's initial dreams seemed to indicate part of his problem regarding his sexual compulsivity. It was a dream in which the split off shadow aspect of the personality that he related to his sexual compulsivity made its first appearance. The dream was as follows:

> Paul is driving a car. A guy wearing a monastic habit with a cowl that made it difficult to see his face is sitting next to him. Paul has an uncomfortable, creepy feeling about this guy and is aware of not wanting to offend him. The man is physically very powerful, like a coiled spring, tense and fidgety. The man moves closer to Paul and he wants to tell him to stay away from him, not to move any closer, but doesn't and plays a non-offensive conciliatory role. Then this guy grabs the wheel and starts to turn the car. He's been waiting to take over and go where he wants to go. Paul doesn't want to go there and tries to keep the car going where he wants to go but can't overpower the man. He awakes with a feeling of fear.

The frightening figure with the cowl and monastic habit represents a personification of a powerful negative shadow aspect in Paul. The dream-ego (that part of the self that is closer to consciousness represented by Paul in the dream) adopts a conciliatory attitude towards this powerful energy and is unable to confront it. Initially, the dream-ego is in control of the personality and is "driving the car," but the shadow figure grabs the wheel and directs the car (representing the personality) where he wants it to go. The dream-ego is left feeling helpless and afraid in the face of this powerful, hostile energy that he feels unable to confront.

Paul's association to the dream was that this man was "criminally insane." He had no conscience, or social correctness; goodness and rightness had no influence over his behavior. *His impulses go unchecked* (emphasis mine) and they are hostile and aggressive. He may do things to hurt others given the chance. Normal restraints would not stop him. He is killer energy. As a personification of the shadow, this man represents powerful energy in the unconscious that has constellated in a negative potentially destructive way. This has occurred because of the repression of instinctual energy and other vital affects. Paul's association to the guy's monastic habit and cowl was that it reminded him of the little people with the electric eyes in Star Wars. They were *impulsive and dangerous* (emphasis mine). Paul associated this man and his energy to his sexually impulsive behavior over which he felt he had no control at times. When this man, representing the split off instinctual sexual energy and affects (Enkidu), took control and grabbed the steering wheel, the ego or more conscious rational left brain aspect of the self (Gilgamesh) was rendered helpless. Paul was able to recognize that he was "a people-pleaser," and that he was frantic to please everyone that he came into contact with. This guy in the dream was aggressive and quite the opposite. Beneath the "nice" self lurked a raw, unformed, primal energy that is crude and abrasive that Paul is afraid to let out. Paul reported that in his family, he was allowed to express only "good" or "nice" feelings. His mother was controlling and very concerned about appearances. She would not tolerate any angry, sad or other "negative" affects. All these affects had to be repressed and relegated to the unconscious. "Niceness" was an important family value, resulting in the development of a people pleasing "nice" false self. It was also everyone's task in the family to keep father happy. So he had to intuit father's feelings and wishes and in this way deny his own needs or desires. This manifested in the transference in his desire to please and entertain me.

Paul was willing to engage with this dream figure in a process of active imagination (as described on p. 148). During this process, the following emerged:

> Dream figure: Nice people threaten me. They don't want me in their world. I am a killer that strangles people.

> Paul: I believe you are very angry and have bottled up your anger for too long.

> Dream figure: When I'm angry, pay attention to me and listen to me. Get out of the way. Don't withdraw behind your pretense of confusion and stuff me back because of what others might think. As the killer, I will protect you but you won't let me do that. You open your abdomen to everyone.

I pointed out that the two of them had to work together to figure this out. Paul agreed. Jung describes the above process of actively engaging an aspect of one's own unconscious as follows:

> He therefore feels compelled, or is encouraged by his analyst, to take part in the play and, instead of just sitting in a theatre, really have it out with his alter ego . . . This process of coming to terms with the Other in us is well worth while, because in this way we get to know aspects of our nature which we would not allow anybody else to show us and which we ourselves would never have admitted. (1963, par. 706)

At this point in the treatment, I introduced Paul to the epic of *Gilgamesh*. He was able to equate the frightening dream figure with Enkidu and his more conscious, rational "nice" false self with Gilgamesh. It seemed clear that part of his inner work was to become more aware of this unconscious "Enkidu energy," to engage with it more consciously and eventually to find a way for these two aspects of his psyche to "become friends."

Jung coined the term *persona* (derived from the Latin word for the mask worn by actors in classical times) to refer to the mask or face with which one confronts the world. Another word to describe this aspect of the personality is the false self. In the gay boy, as the sexual energy is shamed into the unconscious, the stage is set for the development of a compliant, "nice," people pleasing false self or persona. The powerful stream of instinctual sexual libido carries with it not only sexual energy but also access to vital affects (Drescher, 1998a), such as anger, sadness or joy, and the ability to consciously experience the numinous (see above).

In subsequent sessions, Paul reported that the impulse to act out sexually persisted. He had not actually acted out but had engaged in cruising behaviors that had placed him at risk for anonymous sexual encounters. He was however better able to identify when "the addict" (Enkidu, or the man in the cowl in the above dream) was in control. This would occur when he passed an attractive man on the street and turning to see if there was reciprocal interest, looks or touching on the subway, or when visiting places where he had had casual sexual encounters previously. His task was to become more aware of when this "inner addict" was activated and to not allow it to take over control of the personality (that is, to not allow it "to grab the steering wheel of the car," in the language of the above dream).

Paul began to explore more in depth the split that had occurred in his personality. He reported that when he became aware of his same-sex attraction to other little boys in the third grade, he became withdrawn and his lust for life decreased. During adolescence, it was as though someone flipped a switch and the world went dark. He recalled being lonely and miserable during those years and suffering a great deal. Shame and guilt were his constant companions resulting in self-laceration and a sense of inadequacy. Around this time in the treatment, Paul had the following dream:

> A giant was waking up at the bottom of a lake. It was scary. Paul hides behind a wall and hopes that the giant will step over him but is very afraid. Paul did want to see his face though, which was angular. Paul's feeling was that this guy would do exactly as he wanted and wouldn't care what others thought: "It's my way or nothing!"

Paul's association to the giant was that he was strong, powerful, hard and unyielding. This is a somewhat different male energy than in the first dream. Although larger than life and intimidating to the dream-ego, the giant appears to be more benevolent than the guy in the first dream. This indicates that some transformation of the negative masculine energy was occurring in

Paul's psyche. We discussed the similarity of this dream image to the huge, hairy, primitive man that is discovered at the bottom of a pond in the fairy tale of "Iron John." The giant represents in Paul's psyche the despised and repressed positive masculine energy, namely, strength, the willingness to be seen, generativity, clarity and assertiveness. Paul remarked that for him sex represented taking what you wanted when you wanted it. It was thus in his split off sexual activity that Paul could express strength and assertiveness. We wondered together how this energy could be harnessed and expressed in other areas of his life as well.

In the sessions that followed, Paul expressed fears that if he were to say what he was thinking or feeling, that it may hurt me or do damage to me and that I would then reject him. He expressed sadness at his lost sense of wholeness, his loss of a connection with nature and his own inner rhythms. He was beginning to be able to recognize the "damage" to the "bridge" between left and right brain functions, resulting in the shut down of communication between these two aspects of his psyche. Shortly after having the above dream, Paul was able to express some of his angry, despairing affects directly to me as follows:

> I am a bad unworthy person. No one would love me as I am. Jung wasn't able to successfully treat alcoholics. There is nothing that any doctor or medical science in general can do for addicts. The insights are valid but can this stop the acting out? I am scared and desperate. I am mistrustful of you. I don't think that you really believe in sexual addiction and are not educated in treating this problem.

My acceptance of this expression of distrust of me without judgment or retaliation allowed Paul to develop more trust in himself, in me, and in his own process. As our work progressed, Paul began to reflect more on how his cravings for sex were related to his need to be validated for who he is (and this would include his less "nice" more spontaneous self), his need for closeness, and his need to feel worthy and acceptable. He recognized that the more he was able to express his true feelings, the less need he felt to cruise or act out sexually. There was less need to use sex to sedate his discomforting feelings. At my suggestion, he started making crude primitive drawings in order to help him access his inner split off feelings, especially his rage. With the help of a drawing, he was able to let out his rage in a stream of consciousness in one of our sessions as follows:

> Slashing, stabbing rage, murder, aggressor, doing to others what was done to me, like getting back at the whole heterosexual monolithic world. I am raging at the wounding inflicted on us by other men because we are gay. It is other men that enforce this through violence, homophobia, shaming. This has led to a total annihilation of my male

side, of my version of masculinity. How dare they make fun of me, of my "sissy" side, just because I was not like them? The unattainable fantasy of having sex with another man that had to be repressed for so many years: part of my rage is getting even, for being made to feel so one down. Having to repress this rage has led to me being cut off from any spontaneity, so I act out sexually. I feel alive when I act out sexually and I also feel my rage. Under the veneer of people-pleasing is rage. My male energy is very wounded. It is destructive, wounding, betraying, rageful–no warmth, generativity, kindness or empowerment there.

A wounding of the masculine energy because of gender non-conforming behaviors is almost a universal theme that emerges during the course of in-depth psychotherapy with gay men. Drescher points out that boys who grow up to be gay are often gender stressed (1998b, 24). Subsequently, Paul reported that when he was able to connect with his murderous rage and desperation more consciously, the urge to act out sexually decreased. During childhood, he had been afraid that if he expressed his true feelings directly, his parents would withdraw love, he would be abandoned and at risk for dying. He expressed this in the transference relationship with me in the course of our work together, as discussed above. In adulthood, he feared that if he dared to ask for what he needed or expressed his true feelings, something awful would happen or he would be abandoned.

Around this time, Paul had an episode of sexual acting out behavior, and reported feeling heartsick, sad and horrified. I again suggested a process of active imagination in order to engage the "Enkidu energy" and to allow it to have a voice. This is how he expressed himself:

> I like to hide, in the shadows. It is exciting, seeing but not being seen. It is safer. I can leap out at the prey. I like my freedom. Nobody tells me what to do. I can come and go as I want. I don't have to answer to anyone. I like my strength and I live by my senses and wit, listening for sounds of what I can hunt. I am tough and in my prime. I don't have mercy and don't care about others. *Phallus nourishes me, gives me life, makes me feel alive. It's my god, manna, communion, my connection to aliveness, to life . . . survival, food, feeling good. I see myself bringing it to my mouth and just feeding on it. I'll kill anything that gets in the way. I just press it in my mouth and hold it there until I am fed* (emphasis mine). He (referring to the Gilgamesh or intellectual, rational aspect of Paul's psyche) won't let me eat. He stops me because he is a coward. He thinks that the way to survive is by being nice and by not taking what you want. Take the pleasure wherever you can find it and enjoy it, revel in it and don't worry what others think. I starve when he worries about what others think. I feel like a pent-up frightened animal that can't get my food. I'm a great lover. I like sweating and screaming. I'm

hard bone and muscle. I need to run in the forest, to scream with the joy of being free, to say: "I am," to have a voice . . .

I experienced this as a cathartic release of energy that was pouring forth from a deep level of Paul's psyche. It appears from the above that the instinctual or "Enkidu" energy needs the connection with the powerful phallus or Life Force energy in order to be nourished by it. Paul seemed to be connecting with a passion that had all but been extinguished. Something seemed to be shifting for him. He subsequently reported a resurgence of energy and interest in life. It was also becoming easier to identify the shaming voices. It was as though his boundaries had become clearer and he was better able to protect what was important to him. "Gilgamesh" and "Enkidu" seemed to be in the process of at least becoming aware of each other. He reported having close encounters with his inner "Enkidu" but no acting out sexually occurred. He now was better able to converse with "Enkidu" and engage him more consciously. This energy no longer was being allowed to usurp the personality. If he engaged in cruising behaviors, he was able to stay more consciously present during these potential sexual encounters, aware of the risk of disease, of the potential harm to his relationship with his partner and what he'd feel like afterwards. He realized that it was acceptable to feel lonely, sad, horny, unfulfilled. He could just sit with these feelings and did not need to do anything to make them go away. He no longer needed to sedate these affects with sex. He no longer felt compelled to act out sexually.

Paul reported a resurgence of energy in several areas of his life: his work, his creativity, in the relationship with his partner and with his friends. I would like to draw the reader's attention to the above section in italics. This is a spontaneous description of the unconscious "numinous" energy discussed above associated with the phallus. He reported that his sex life with his partner had also improved. He was aware at times of experiencing powerful truly primal sexual energies when making love with his partner. Sometimes it felt as though he just wanted to worship his partner's phallus. The split off numinous energy, formerly projected onto the phallus of strangers where it was worshipped, was beginning to be experienced in the context of the relationship with his partner. The excitement affect, formerly only experienced in the context of anonymous sexual encounters, was also being experienced while making love with his partner.

Paul has not had any further sexual encounters that he would regard as sexually compulsive behavior for the past several months. He continues to struggle with the "Enkidu" energy that still at times wants to usurp the personality and take over. However, he is now better able to express most of his feelings more appropriately, including the not so "nice" ones, and no longer needs sex to sedate them. He has discussed his awareness that he can celebrate his life in ways that are not only sexual. He is beginning to be aware that the numinous can be experienced in other circumstances as well. He is learning to "celebrate" (that is, connect with the numinous) through creativity and is giving himself time to express this. He is aware that he can experience the numinous in ways that do not only have to be "exciting," such as the joy of being in nature, the pleasure of listening to music and the enjoyment of being more present in his body. He is also beginning to experience this numinous energy in his sexual expression with his partner. It would seem that the "Gilgamesh" and "Enkidu" aspects of his psyche at least have a working relationship now, even if they are not as yet "the best of friends." The "bridge" which allows for a free interchange of energy between left and right hemispheres of the brain is becoming more functional. His awareness of these powerful energies in his inner world and how they influence his life, his willingness to engage them, as well as his ability to accept his limitations and strengths, may allow him to acquire wisdom. That was the final outcome of the quest of Gilgamesh. He ultimately had to accept the reality of his own humanity and mortality. He came to accept the pain of the loss of his beloved friend, Enkidu, and finally returned to Uruk to rule as king. It is as a result of this acceptance of our own humanity and lot in life that we become wiser and can participate in the joy of living our lives as fully as possible.

CONCLUSION

It is impossible to convey the complexity of what occurs when two people are working at a depth level with the powerful forces of the psyche. I have only focussed on relevant material in my work with Paul in order to illustrate my particular way of working within a Jungian framework. The material I have presented was selected to illustrate the split that occurs in many gay men between intellect and instinct, left and right brain hemispheres, as a result primarily of shaming related to homosexual impulses and gender non-conforming behaviors. This profoundly affects the ability to have intimate relationships in which empathic connection and sexuality can co-exist in the context of a love relationship. It was my intention to illustrate not only that sexual energy is split off and repressed in the unconscious but many other vital affects as well. I wished to illustrate the connection between sexuality and "numinous" experiences and this also influenced my selection of clinical material. Working with the intrapsychic energies as they initially constellated in Paul's psyche, by actively engaging them and observing their capacity to transform from one form to another, I hoped to illustrate a teleological approach to psychotherapy. However, I also incorporated aspects of Paul's childhood, his family relationships, and his interactions with peers when important to the overall treatment process. I am deeply indebted to Paul and all those who grant me the privilege of facilitating their processes.

BIBLIOGRAPHY

Drescher, J. (1998a), Contemporary psychoanalytic psychotherapy with gay men with a commentary on reparative therapy of homosexuality. *J. Gay & Lesbian Psychotherapy*, 2(4): 51-74.

_____ (1998b), *Psychoanalytic Therapy and the Gay Man*. Hillsdale: The Analytic Press.

Edinger, E. (1985), *Anatomy of the Psyche*. La Salle, IL: Open Court, 72.

Eliade, M. (1969), *Images and Symbols*. New York: Sheed and Ward.

Jung, C.G. (1950), The Symbolic Life. *The Collected Works of C.G. Jung*, Princeton: Princeton University Press, Vol. 18.

_____ (1954), The Practice of Psychotherapy. *The Collected Works of C.G. Jung*, Princeton: Princeton University Press, Vol. 16.

_____ (1956), Symbols of Transformation. *The Collected Works of C.G. Jung*, Princeton: Princeton University Press, Vol. 5.

_____ (1958), Psychology and Religion. *The Collected Works of C.G. Jung*, London: Routledge & Kegan Paul, Vol. 11.

_____ (1963), Mysterium Coniunctionis. *The Collected Works of C.G. Jung*, New York: Princeton University Press, Vol. 14.

Kaufman, G., Raphael, L. (1996), *Coming Out of Shame*. New York: Doubleday.

Mason, H. (1970), *Gilgamesh*. New York and Scarborough, Ontario: New American Library.

Monick, E. (1987), *Phallos: Sacred Image of the Masculine*. Toronto: Inner City Books.

Otto, R. (1926), *The Idea of the Holy*. London: Oxford University Press.

Otto, W. (1965), *Dionysus Myth and Cult*. Bloomington, IN: University of Indiana Press.

Samuels, A., Shorter, B., & Plaut, F. (1986), *A Critical Dictionary of Jungian Analysis*. London and New York: Routledge & Kegan Paul.

Scasta, D. (1998), Issues in helping people come out. *J. Gay & Lesbian Psychotherapy*, 2(4): 87-98.

Winnicott, D.W. (1960), Ego distortion in terms of true and false self, in *The Maturational Processes and the Facilitating Environment*. (1965). New York: International University Press, 140-152.

Vanggaard, Thorkkil. (1972), *Phallos*. New York: Universities Press, Inc.

APPENDIX
PAUL'S RESPONSE

I have read much about what causes, perpetuates, and triggers sexual addiction and am deeply committed to a twelve-step recovery program. Even so, remaining sexually sober in the face of addictive fantasies and impulses has been difficult and often takes considerable effort. I am not alone in this. I see many in my sexual addiction recovery program also struggling to maintain basic abstinence from their bottom-line addictive behaviors. I have found the Jungian-oriented, eclectic psychotherapy that John offers effective in strengthening my abstinence and sobriety.

For me, the most important aspect of working with John has been the building of a relationship where my trust and sense of safety were sufficient to expose and explore my real feelings and thoughts. This in turn enabled me to risk experiencing and expressing feelings in a different way. The safety of the container created in our therapeutic work itself became the catalyst for the change and healing I sought. The building of this container took a long time. A critical step in this process occurred when I realized that John was not going to shame my sexuality or me, when I understood emotionally that he was focused on helping me to stop shaming myself. This taught me the value of a therapist who has dealt with his own issues. Though this is something we never discussed directly, I believe that John could only have provided this safe place for me by first working through his own sexual shame.

In the safe space provided by the container of my therapy sessions, I was able to experience the realities described by the affect theory presented in the first section of this paper. I sought to act out sexually as a way to medicate the momentary shame, fear, and anxiety arising from specific situations or triggers in my life. In the course of my therapy, I learned I could both tolerate and endure these emotions in the moment without a catastrophe happening. Also, I learned how to soothe myself and release or counteract these feelings so that they didn't persist or escalate. Through therapy, I came to know that I also used sexual acting out behaviors to punish both others and myself. Acting out expressed the rage I felt towards men in general, my father in particular, and the deep and painful oppression of the monolithic heterosexist world perpetrated on gay men. I learned that underneath fantasies of sexually acting out lay a craving for attention, affection, and affirmation–a craving that I could meet better in other ways. I realized that addictive sex was a way of rewarding myself with excitement and passion.

Addictive sex was also the dark way I experienced a sense of the holy–a sense of truly being alive. I began to allow myself to experience passion and holiness in healthier ways in other areas of my life, specifically in my relationship with my partner, my creative life, my work, and my contact with nature. An experience that happened on a hike sums this up for me. Hearing an eerie cry, I peered into the mist of a sheltered arm of the sea and saw a merganser, free and wild, lifting its open beak into the mist and singing with a sort of ecstasy. Feelings awoke in me of aliveness and passion deeper and much more satisfying than those I felt momentarily when acting out sexually. And unlike acting out, I could remember and recount this experience without releasing a torrent of shame!

Recovery from sexual addiction has not meant making my sex life unimportant, but instead has led to it becoming important in different ways. The worship of the phallus comes naturally to me. The shameful, fearful part of me cringes as I write this; however, there is nothing I like better than taking my partner's hard cock in my mouth and bringing him to orgasm. It is fully equal to the pleasure of my own orgasm and seems something at once intimate and cosmic and wholly engrossing. I believe that allowing myself to have this experience with my partner helps release psychic energies, the knotting and cross-wiring of which results in compulsive sexual acting out.

I relate to the worship of the phallus primarily through the notion of spirituality. It means that sex with my partner and the sexual dimension of my interactions with others and the world at large becomes a gateway for vitality, meaning, the free flow of feeling, the experience of wholeness, and connection with the divine. My ability to regard sucking cock as a legitimate form of worship stretches my conception of the spiritual. When I think of this, I hear a stern and punitive voice say: "Thou shalt worship no other gods before me." But is this God speaking or William Blake's Nobodaddy? The Self in Jungian terms (God, wholeness) does not preempt the archetypes but flows in and through them and their interactions. Perhaps it can be best said that the archetypes and their interactions exist in and because of the Self. However I conceptualize this in theory or in my therapeutic work, seeing hot sex with my partner as a worshipful act opens me to experience spiritual energy, serves as an antidote to sexual shame, and is healing. So I have welcomed this idea, trying neither to cling to it heavy-handedly nor to look to it as yet another way of medicating uncomfortable feelings.

I found the Jungian bent of our therapy sessions helpful. The many vivid dreams I had during our therapeutic work served as guideposts or trail markers on my journey, windows into the deep workings of my soul. They shed light on the progress I had made and the work that was yet to be done. Likewise, working with active imagination and fantasy during sessions and bringing in artwork I created between sessions helped me connect with the creative power and wisdom of my psyche. Exploring mythological analogues to my struggles not only gave me insight into them and metaphors to help me in my daily struggle with addiction, it made me feel less alone–people in other times and cultures have struggled with these same issues. John's involvement and guidance in this process were essential. I was as apt to interpret a dream out of my perfectionism and shame, for instance, as out of connection with my deeper center. When the perfectionism and shame became active in the symbolic work, John extended a firm hand to help me observe them and choose another way.

In our sessions, I was able to face to some extent my fear of death, the great linchpin that keeps the cycle of shame and anxiety fueled and running like a juggernaut. John helped me peek beneath the surface of this fear and emotionally experience death simply as a part of life. I believe he could only do this because he has to some extent dealt with his own fear of death.

Finally, the experience of reading the drafts of this article and adding to it has been a powerful healing experience. It has helped me understand the place I started from, where I am now and why I feel healthier. Through it, I appreciate how far I have come and how far I still have to go.

Reification and the Ecstasy of the Chelsea Boy

Stephen Hartman, PhD

SUMMARY. This essay describes the convergence of psychological and political experience in gay men's development of subjectivity. It explores a process whereby gay men recognize themselves to be gay like other gays and articulate their individual way of being gay through this act of recognition. *Reification* is introduced to describe the gay subject's encounter with objectified gayness–a task of individuation that is often overlooked. The psycho-political space where these acts of recognition and individuation occur is called "Chelsea space," here, so as to offer a way of thinking about substance use among urban, gay "Chelsea Boys." Case material is woven through the essay, and different degrees of substance use are understood to reflect different uses of the subject/object encounter that occurs in Chelsea space. *[Article copies available for a fee from The Haworth Document Delivery Service: 1-800-342-9678. E-mail address: <getinfo@haworthpress inc.com> Website: <http://www.HaworthPress.com>]*

KEYWORDS. Homosexuality, substance abuse, reification, psychoanalytic theory, gay substance abusers, recognition, Chelsea Boys

Maybe you believe people are born gay, or maybe you don't. Maybe you assume that we are born with a biologically assigned gender. Or maybe you would argue that gender is a culturally assigned, socially constructed category. Perhaps these are not questions that you worry much about. (I have long thought that knowing the answer to these questions is less important than

Dr. Stephen Hartman is a Clinical Psychologist, New York, NY, and a Postdoctoral Candidate in Psychotherapy and Psychoanalysis, New York University.

[Haworth co-indexing entry note]: "Reification and the Ecstasy of the Chelsea Boy." Hartman, Stephen. Co-published simultaneously in *Journal of Gay & Lesbian Psychotherapy* (The Haworth Medical Press, an imprint of The Haworth Press, Inc.) Vol. 3, No. 3/4, 2000, pp. 169-185; and: *Addictions in the Gay and Lesbian Community* (ed: Jeffrey R. Guss, and Jack Drescher) The Haworth Medical Press, an imprint of The Haworth Press, Inc., 2000, pp. 169-185. Single or multiple copies of this article are available from The Haworth Document Delivery Service [1-800-342-9678, 9:00 a.m. - 5:00 p.m. (EST). E-mail address: getinfo@haworthpressinc.com].

© 2000 by The Haworth Press, Inc. All rights reserved.

understanding why they are so persistently raised.) Still, if you found your-self at a magazine stand and a cover picture of two GLBT icons (Greg Louganis and Alexandra Billings) jumped out at you, how might you respond to the banner headlines THIS MAN WAS BORN GAY. THIS WOMAN WAS BORN MALE.[1] Proud? Curious? Dubious? It's likely that your re-sponse depends on what you believe about sexuality and gender, where you are when you spot the *Advocate* (where it appeared), your comfort with the inclusion of transgender issues in gay and lesbian politics, and whether or not you understand how the image is being used editorially. You also can appreci-ate that the cover sells the magazine (it's catchy in an "I got all my sisters with me" way). So, you might not care much about the "born gay" slogan, and you might just smile.

Now compare the image of our own Greg and Alexandra with the familiar photograph of John and Anne Paulk. As the poster children of the Ex-Gay movement, the Paulks appeared on the cover of *Newsweek* and were seen in many major news magazines in the spring of 1999. The posed Paulks bring to mind an awareness of stubborn homophobia–stubborn in current political life and, maybe, in your past experience. Suppose a magazine cover featuring the Paulks was on the shelf next to one with the born-gay icons. And suppose you were on the fence about the "born gay" issue. Let's say you had just heard of Matthew Shepard's murder or watched a film where Teena Brandon's humili-ations were brutally depicted. Might you in an emotional moment consent (*we are born gay!*) because you were feeling something political?

If the image of Louganis and Billings or the Paulks piques some political awareness for you, I would venture to guess that it also has personal resonance. In this essay, I want to describe a space where the political and psychological converge. Just as we each have our own "subjective" experience of being gay, there are times, like when the Paulks nosey into our lives, when we realize that gayness is also an objectified political category. I use the term "objectified" to state strongly that when political discourse enters our personal space, we meet gayness as a *thing* that people do or don't have rather than as an experience that people pursue and shape according to their own desires and needs. (Do you have that gay gene? Do you live that gay lifestyle?) Think about it this way: you probably already knew what "faggot" or "lezzie" meant the first time you were called one. Before we are even aware that such a thing as identity exists (a patient wisely told me), we have *it*. For reasons that I will get to in a moment, I believe we need to keep this idea of gayness as "thing" in mind when thinking about substance use in our community. My hope is to describe certain substance use practices in a political and psychological space where one recognizes and wrangles with objectified gayness. It is a psycholog-ical space not unlike standing in a magazine shop, staring at our born-gay heroes and the ex-gay Paulks and, in a moment of recognition, concurring, "Born gay!" or thinking, "That is me."

The gay thing predates us. Just as we're born with parents who lend us our genetic imprint and influence our developmental path so, too, are we "born gay." There is an always already there Gayness (that first appellation "faggot" in relation to which we are "a gay object"). We meet ourselves as gay objects en route to finding our own way of being gay. To borrow a Lacanian precept, "the human animal is born into language and it is within the terms of language that the human subject is constructed. Language does not arise from within the individual, it is always out there in the world outside, lying in wait for the neonate" (J. Mitchell, 1982, p. 5). And, after Foucault, we can add that the terms "faggot" and "lezzie" await us *and* discipline us. We are compelled to take a stand (come out) in order to be gay, so our quest for self-efficacy takes a political shape. Perhaps the power of the *Advocate* headline is to evoke an uncomplicated, certain gayness in a moment of preordained doubt: is *that* me?

From this vantage, "born gay" or "born male" is an ideal of being like (gay) others even before being told that we are not like (straight) others. It is an objectification (as if gayness were a thing) and an appropriation of hetero-sexist binaries but also a set of terms and categories that we use to represent ourselves to ourselves and to others. On some important but difficult to understand level, we all have to contend with our objectified selves in order to be gay in ways that distinguish us as gay individuals. Where you go when you walk away from the newsstand is up to you.

Individuation (that is, developing a subjectivity among like and different others) within the context of a politicized, objectified identity is a complex problem. Psychoanalytic inquiry has not paid a great deal of attention to the burden of objectification for members of minority communities. How do we meet ourselves already objectified? Is this encounter one that we sometimes need to revisit in the way that we might reenact some moment in our relationship with early caretakers?

Here is a contradiction to reckon with: sometimes I, and I imagine all of us, need a break from being Gay–from being gay by investiture–from being what others (straight and gay) imagine the born-gay are like. I want to move in a more subjective space that tenders my own desires. Oddly enough, I typically find it in the thick of gay life: my favorite outdoor cafe bench on Chelsea's Eighth Avenue strip, the gym, a foreign gay beach where I eye men with a sense of seamless alikeness. In these almost stereotypical spaces I am both subjectively and objectively gay at the same time. I do the gay thing in gay quarters, but I do it my way. I enter what Bollas (1992, p. 18, developing an idea put forth by Winnicott) calls *intermediate space*, "the space where subject meets thing, to confer significance in the very moment that being is transformed by the object." A transformation takes place and I am at once born-gay and gay by my own design. My need for personal space was recognized and met in gay public space. So, in the space where I initially sought a break from being Dr. Gay, I found myself being a gay object doing stereotypically gay things. Most importantly, I was doing gay things among other gay objects and, in recognizing that object relation, and feeling the power of my own desires, I became a gay subject. Here, "subject" has two shades of meaning: I experience my otherness (not straight) while also feeling my own subjective desires.

I want to theorize the psychological and political space where many gay men encounter themselves as a gay object. This is an experience that is superadded to the necessary task of becoming a person in relation to other persons. It is a process that, I believe, anyone who says they are "gay" confronts, but a process that gets realized in different ways—some more difficult than others. Here, I will mostly concern myself with gay substance abusers who, in the context of psychotherapy, relate their drug use to a wish for a comfortable, objectified space of gayness. I will ponder what psychodynamic work takes place there and, again, in its retelling in psychotherapy.

Many gay men whom I meet use drugs to retrieve a subjective sense of gayness while "doing the gay thing." It is a paradox, but, to use my metaphor from earlier, when they eye Greg and Alexandra there is a rush of familiarity and confidence that comforts feelings of self-contempt or estrangement: I am the thing that the Paulks most fear. Among a certain gay type, the drug-addicted "Chelsea Boy,"[2] this process of recognizing and articulating subjectivity while dabbling in objectified zones is highly problematic because of its connection to repeated drug use. I have found that many gay substance abusers react against the essentializing strictures of the Paulk's "homosexuality," just like non-addicts, by embracing a space of sameness with other gay men. Somehow, in the cloned space of reduced subjectivity, subjectivity emerges from feeling oneself an object among like objects. Sadly, for drug-addicted individuals, this occurs in a dangerous, chemically altered state in which subjective desires amalgamate more intensely than they individuate. On drugs like ecstasy or cocaine, bonding with other Chelsea Boys may be fast but the process of recognizing one's own subjective desire separate from objectified forms of desire is slowed down. More troublesome, addiction is a space that repeats relations of dependence on forces that would define you.

*   *   *   *   *

To locate drug dependence in psycho-political space, I have borrowed the term *reification* from Marxist theory (Lukacs, 1971).[3] Reification was the term Marx used to describe the state of affairs when social relations between men, the experience of work in particular, appeared to assume the form of a relation between things–owners of capital and laborers. If we think of reification in a psychoanalytic frame, reification deals with the way that apparently objective categories that describe social relations are taken into subjective experience. Reification is a more political concept than its psychoanalytic cousin, "internalization," and a more spatial one because it describes how we rank our internal sense of ourselves in power relations to others. Reified gayness is not only an internal sense of homosexual orientation but, also, an internalized sense that gayness stands in a seemingly objective, binary relation to "normal" heterosexuality. Psychologically, then, reification entails the individual's encoding and internalization of already-reified political categories. As Fuss (1991, p. 3) explains, "Heterosexuality can never fully ignore the close psychical proximity of its terrifying (homo)sexual other, any more than homosexuality can entirely escape the equally insistent pressures of (hetero)sexual conformity." Awareness of reification occurs in spaces of recognizing the "thing" status of aspects of self, for example, "Born Gay" at the magazine stand. It prompts us to think about the way that human experience becomes structured in categories that are seemingly "objective" as a consequence of social and linguistic practices.

In my view, gays and lesbians are constrained to identify themselves using reified categories of sexual difference (from heterosexual norms) as the basis of anything they may say about themselves as gay individuals. Take the coming out story as an example. Elsewhere, I demonstrated how this quintessential gay story becomes an identity performance space for gay storytellers (Hartman, 1995).[4] A coming out story follows a fairly standard format or *fabula*: it identifies the speaker as someone who was "in the closet," then struggled with some aspect of desire and identity, then decided to come out to someone whom he told he was gay and, then, went on to be gay–as telling the story demonstrates. However, gay speakers who tell coming out stories, must apply categories of experience that do not necessarily feel their own. They thwart the standard *fabula* by adding idiosyncratic stylistic and plot turns in order to tell the story in a way that renders it their own. The point is that regularly, as gay men and women, we are compelled to describe ourselves in categories that are given to us in the form of an already-there identity in order to have a voice. We may have unhappy associations to the spaces where those categories were first recognized (e.g., the school playground) and we may have earlier, "unconscious" associations with those categories that take us back to early years of life. But we still use those categories. They place us as "gay" in a definite but malleable relation to others who are "straight."

An interesting thing about telling a coming out story retrospectively is that it occurs in a space where narrator and listener both recognize the story's standard *fabula* yet focus on the speaker's particular experience. It is as though being "gay" is less at issue than how the storyteller did it. With little thought, we recognize how something objectified can also be something personal or "subjectified." For Marxist thinkers, work (as the spatial zone of alienated labor) was where this could happen. For many psychoanalytic thinkers, this "space" where self meets its constituent structures, is the transference-countertransference relationship. For many gay men, one meets his objectified self in Chelsea.

*   *   *   *   *

In a world where people have multiple possibilities for what they might be, Chelsea Boys might be seen to have a kind of "variable self" (S. Mitchell, 1993). Organized in different ways at different times, there is no one way to be a Chelsea Boy. Nor does being a Chelsea Boy some of the time mean being a Chelsea Boy all the time. "Oh my, I see we are in High Chelsea today!" a patient recently commented on meeting me in the street wearing cargo pants and a tank top. The Chelsea Boy is a way of presenting oneself that is "variable" because it "appears as multiple patterns grounded in different, prototypical interactions with others." If by day I experience myself to be a banker, by night I may go home to Chelsea and don leather. In either case, being located in an object relation to "Chelsea" is to be gay among like others. (Louis says, "I leave the bank, and after feeling like my HIV status is a big secret all day, I just want to be somewhere where it's nothing. Even though I live uptown, I walk to Chelsea to catch the subway." Greg, a publicist, says: "I don't know what it is. I get off the plane after visiting my mom and I head straight to Splash! It's not like I'm some kind of Chelsea queen! I never go to Splash. But after a weekend at home, I feel compelled to be surrounded by gay boys.") Sometimes these patterns are stereotypical: a readily identifiable look; a certain lifestyle. But, in reality, the Chelsea Boy experience is a form of membership in the urban, gay cosmos and a highly subjective experience. One opts for it as a particular kind of self-experience on an as-needed basis. One doesn't ultimately need the paraphernalia or the attitude, just a wish to relate to other gay men in a characteristic way.

How one relates to others reflects on how one places oneself among various possibilities for what one might be. The Chelsea Boy is a complex construction made up of many such possibilities. Louis and Greg (above) see Chelsea as a place or, we might say, an identity space that fits certain needs. It allows for a certain type of self-experience and a certain type of comfort. The idea that people relate in profound ways to diverse aspects of themselves is relatively recent in psychoanalysis. Bollas (1987) argued that each person's self is the history of several internal relations (e.g., son, adult, gay man, banker, Chelsea Boy, analysand, etc.). We experience aspects of self-experience through the interplay of internal and external reality:

Once any one part is objectified (in thought or in feeling) it thereupon comes into existence. There is no one unified mental phenomenon that we can term self . . . Over a lifetime we objectify, know and 'relate to' the many different states in our being. Emotional and psychological realities bring with them self-states, which become parts of our history. The concept of self should refer to the positions or points of view from which and through which we sense, feel, observe and reflect on distinct and separate experiences in our being. One crucial point of view comes through the other who experiences us. (pp. 9-10)

Indeed, we are sons and adults and bankers and Chelsea Boys in relation to others and in relation to what we understand about ourselves. For Bollas, we often place ourselves in spaces that cast us in a relation to experiences that we need to revisit or rework. (Think about Chelsea Boys at the gym.)[5] The work of dealing with conflictual self-relations takes place in particular spaces and, often, in the form of "moods." A kind of "experience memory" preserves states of being that are linked to the child self's continuing negotiation with some aspect of the early parental care environment. These important experiences are linked to moods that may or may not be readily understood. People from our past may reside in certain of our moods where the mood signifies our relationship to them and to a way of being ourselves. "Malignant moods" can be read as reactions against another object–a kind of stymied self-space where it is not possible to recognize the feelings and interpersonal experiences that the mood recalls. By contrast, in a more dialogic, "generative mood," Bollas believes that a person goes into the mind of the "mute, unknown child self and thus has a greater chance of generating some knowing of what has been part of the unthought known" (p. 101).

Chelsea, as I am conceptualizing it, is a mood space where one visits reified categories of gayness among others who resemble you. In Chelsea space, we go into the mind of heterosexism's other. In our culture that essentializes homosexuality to sustain its distinct difference from heterosexuality, the Chelsea Boy inhabits a kind of gay playground. The Chelsea Boy appears to be stripped of subjectivity (as the clone form of 90s Homo) yet, in reality, he is laden with the multiple possibilities for *whatever* performance of gayness. There really is no such thing as a Chelsea Boy per se. There are many versions of Chelsea Boy. It is a thing, though, that gay men can fashion, fantasize or, even, fetishize. And to use Bollas' metaphor, it is a space that can be relatively "generative" or "malignant" along a continuum of investments in being there. Whether the space being a Chelsea Boy provides allows a person to emerge as a distinct personality or to blend without distinction depends, largely, on the person's relative ability (and desire) to individuate from reified gayness.

I am suggesting that a person who has a problematic relationship to the reified "gay thing" profits from recognizing that other Chelsea Boys share a similar experience. Chelsea has rituals that are importantly social, public and highly visible. There is a Chelsea Boy in stereotype form: goes to the gym, eats and shops on Eighth Avenue, works out and achieves a desirable body; parties in large crowds at circuit parties, uses cocaine, ecstasy, special K; has sexual adventures one after the next with other beautiful Chelsea Boys. Chelsea Boys often share the fantasy, described most recently by Mendelsohn (1999, p. 6), of social self-discovery: "I secretly imagined a place where all the people were other boys and where all the stories and books and songs and movies and restaurants were by boys about other boys. It would be a place where somehow the outside reality of the world that met your eyes and ears could finally be made to match the inner, hidden reality of what you knew yourself to be." In this idealized forum of gayness, Chelsea space provides others who are like oneself for an experiment in self-acceptance, not unlike Freud's ego-ideal.

Freud developed the concept of ego-ideal in his 1914 essay *On Narcissism*. As Benjamin (1998) explains, he proposed that we either love a "maternal" other who is our source of care and protection, or we love someone who represents a part of ourselves that we once were, would like to be, maybe know we cannot be. The relationship to the ego-ideal, what Benjamin calls "identificatory love," had been seen as characteristic of narcissism (because it inhibits appreciation of others' subjective difference),[6] but it need not be. Benjamin explores the power of recognition at work when we relate to love objects who are like subjects:

> When we recognize the outside other as a separate and equivalent center of subjectivity, she is a "like subject." When, on the other hand, we identify with the other as inner representation, taking the other as the ideal of who we might wish to become, we also set up a relation of "like subjects." (p. 7)

For Benjamin, mutual recognition preserves a necessary tension of independence/dependence between subjects that allows for autonomy and differentiation. I would add that, in a context where subjectivity is mired in reifying forces, where there is an allure to being "born gay" like others so that one can get on with being oneself, we have a need to recognize that other gay men and women also wrangle with a reified, objectified subjectivity. In other words, we play out "the gay thing" among others who are like us, and we recognize that we need not be *that* thing—or, if we do wish to be like that, it is a personal choice. To take on this trying task, many gay men place themselves in Chelsea space. Once there, some use drugs repeatedly to the point that they experience neither subjectivity nor autonomy—but addiction.

Benjamin wisely points out that recognition of this type is a capacity of individual development that is "only unevenly realized" because it is necessarily destabilizing. She notes (p. 37) that "at the very moment we come to understand the meaning of I, *myself,* we are forced to see the limitations of that self because we depend upon another to recognize it." For gay children, in the heterosexual care environment, such recognition may not be readily available (Frommer, 1994; Isay, 1989). And the task of recognizing oneself among others who might be like us often takes an ugly turn. In the space of "the closet"[7] we relate to others via intrapsychic fears that we, and others like us, will be destroyed. It is not surprising, then, that some men take Chelsea at its worst. To be caught up in addiction is to be caught in a malignant mood, a space where others drift in as like shadows of an unrelated self. As Benjamin understands, when the other's reality does not come into view, aggression against like subjects is internalized in self-destructive fantasy: there is "the loss of balance between the intrapsychic and the intersubjective, between fantasy and reality" (p. 40). In the closet as in its residual spaces, the heterosexual/homosexual binary is reified to the extent that experiences of self are all but eradicated.

*   *   *   *   *

The experience of self also appears to be eradicated in addiction. If recreational drug use and other Chelsea rituals provide a sensation of autonomy for some men, this experience must be contrasted to addiction. In addiction, objectified rituals are repeated with a decreasing sense of autonomy, increased dependence on repeating these rituals, and a convergence of self-experience with use. (Aaron says: "I had no responsibilities when I was using, no relationships. The only thing I had to do was keep getting drugs. That was all I did. There was no me making decisions.") Of course, forging a distinction about "normal" and "pathological" drug use is a quagmire, and I don't wish to get bogged down in an effort to identify acceptable use. Rather than focus on quantitative measures of use, I want to focus on relative degrees of autonomy in the self-experience that I have heard people (casual users and self-proclaimed "addicts") report. Let's begin with the literary description of ecstasy-born reverie in Alan Hollinghurst's *The Spell* (1998, p. 85). Alex, a rather frigid civil servant, has taken ecstasy for the first time:

> They were dancing in the middle of the floor, in a loose group with some other friends of Danny's. Alex had never felt so agile or so energized. He pulled off his wet T-shirt, and knew what a shinning streak of sinewy beauty he was from the way people looked at him and lightly touched him. His thick black hair was soaked, and fell forward and was flung back. He danced like everyone else now, but better, more remarkably. He found himself staring rapturously at the dancers around him–it was never deliberate, it was as if he woke up to find his gaze locked with a grinning stranger's.

Alex's reverie is bounded by his desire to commune with like subjects. It is a desire that has been long repressed and is awoken when (through a new boyfriend) he finds himself in a dancing crowd of boys on drugs. He experiences the frisson of flirtation as if it were total contact. When not using, he distinguishes this buoyant feeling from the more enduring sense of love.[8] (Ahmed says: "it's silly fun to be part of it all and to dance and laugh without worrying about who you are or who anyone else is.") Arguably, Alex dances himself Gay: the experience of being in a crowd of gay men helps him to be comfortable with areas of self-doubt. These doubts are present in the many aspects of his civil servant life where he juggles his subjective likes and dislikes with a sense of needing to self-censure and conform to the straight world's way. He believes, whether or not it is true, that he got to this liberating communal space because of the disinhibiting and pleasure heightening effects of ecstasy. Be that as it may, Hollinghurst casts Alex's visit to (what I'm calling) Chelsea space as a kind of wake up call to gay self-awareness.

A patient who I mentioned earlier, Greg, recently asked me if I thought his love of dancing shirtless in the beefy circuit party swarm was something to be ashamed of: on one hand, it feels so enlivening; on the other, he worried, "so unevolved." Greg hopes that I will recognize this contradiction, as I myself am gay. And my recognizing this contradiction seems to serve as witness to my recognizing something important about Greg. He says, a week later, "It's bizarre, some of the things I let myself say to you! You could really judge me for it. And yet, when I tell you about it, it feels like it's understandable to want to have sex or share a bump with some boy I just met. I like just being able to say anything for that reason."

For Greg, occasional drug use or casual sex provides a sense of permission to be gay and to be free from his family's expectations. Greg came to therapy because he was concerned that his siblings were all married while he, gay and single at 42, seemed to have no prospects. Greg grew up in a large, status conscious, Northern California family. When his father died (Greg, the oldest child, was 38), Greg became the family member whose duty it was to remind his siblings of their familial obligations. Even before his father's death, Greg was aware that he played some significant role in the family's efforts after the appearance of stability. He had a sense of being called upon, also, to defer his sexual development for the family. He recalls difficulty coming out or settling into his first long-term relationship against the backdrop of his perception that being gay would have a destabilizing effect on the family.

Greg's reified self experience is sufficiently "recognized" in Chelsea space that it can be comfortably elaborated upon in his own musings and explored in the intersubjective space of psychotherapy. Greg uses the "transference" space to express the experience of feeling objectified: as judged by someone who might attack his desires and, also, as alike with his gay therapist. He gathers a sense of autonomy through Chelsea rituals that is often fleeting, and he uses therapy both to consolidate a sense of autonomy and to understand how, in many aspects of his experience that challenge his autonomy, he is himself.

In the most serious addictions, if there is a sense of union with like "subjects" or alternative experiences of self, it is typically a meeting among "things"–reified objects that have fleeting or unstable experience of like subjectivity. If I am smoking crack with other crackheads, in other words, I am not relating to people. Their "heads" don't matter to me. Mine, as Aaron said earlier, is only focused on getting more drugs. I'm "on a run" but I'm standing still when it comes to elaborating my desires. In serious addiction, then, the subjectifying experience of meeting oneself reified either does not occur or it does not influence self-experience outside the ritualized context of drug use. The kinds of difference (not straight) that are similar (Gay) in Chelsea space are dramatically reduced and paired down to very basic elements. Here is Jeremy's description of this space: "I only smoke cocaine in a group where everyone there is as 'no one' as me. You find out about it in a chat room on the web. Someone is looking for 'a group of guys to party' and you know it'll be *that*. I hate myself like *that* but, when I'm in the head to use, it doesn't matter. I want to be with those people even though I know I have no business being there." Aaron adds how sex, too, is selfless, other-less and "that" in this space: "Everyone at the sex club is coked up. If someone approaches me and shows any sign of recognizing me or wanting to know me, I look at them with a look like 'wrong! That's not how it is here.' Everyone there is supposed to know that. It's a big part of the experience."

As I mentioned earlier, the wish for a comfortable space in which to experience identification with like subjects may not be available to all gay men. Jeremy, for one, hates desiring "like that" yet can't see his way around it. Recalling Bollas' distinction, if for some men the encounter with peers whose sexual identity is similarly reified is "generative," for others, it has a "malignant" quality:

> In my view, what differentiates a generative from a malignant mood is that nature of the mood's function and the quality of that boundary that preserves a space for mood experiencing. If we feel, let's say, that a person's withdrawn imperviousness is a means of coercing another into serving some self function, then such a mood would constitute a malignant interpersonal process, one which I would like to differentiate from generative withdrawal, when we do not feel that the person's mood is fundamentally aimed to force us into some captitulative activity. (1987, pp. 100-101)

For Jeremy and Aaron, Chelsea space is well known and often sought, but any recognition that happens in that space is neither understood nor assimilated into a more complex view of self and other. In this malignant space, people are there to use like fuel for the keep-running drug engine. Furthermore, as was particularly evident in Aaron's statement, other Chelsea Boys' experience of self is assumed to be as voided as one's own and, arguably, others are only allowed into Chelsea space to demonstrate that seeming fact. There is a sense of identification, being among other gay men for sex or drugs, but little or no sense of who those men are distinct from the fact that they participate in similar desire. I am not saying that these men are merely used to mirror feelings of emptiness; it is critical that they be (at least in that moment) on drugs and Gay where gay equals *"that is how it is here."*

Furthermore, these men use highly addictive substances that they abuse to the point of dependence. As Aaron says, "how *it* is here," i.e., being with others who observe the rituals of use, is what they depend on. There is no generative or dialogic "boundary" to "preserve a space for mood experiencing." No one can provide a sufficient sense of a mood (or self) other than *that.* No friend, sponsor, therapist, parent or lover is independent enough of homophobia to grant a true feeling of reprieve from the persistent struggle: use, shame, rehabilitation, relapse, try again. The addict's limited use of Chelsea space (to find Like separate from Other without experiencing difference) reflects a problem in the ability to grant anyone independence from reified roles and to feel independent in turn. Note that it is a property of chemical dependency that drug use repeats relations of dependence on forces that define you. In repeated use, addiction feels as powerful and defining as heterosexuality and, like heterosexual/homosexual relations, it overwhelms. For Jeremy and Aaron, drug use has been ritualized to the point that it exerts a stranglehold on any differentiation that might take place in alternative, non-drug related Chelsea spaces. The experience of self as distinct from use, then, is at best fleeting: enough to yearn for, yet not enough to engender autonomy. Chelsea space simply provides this: being around other people who experience themselves as a drug using, sexing *it*, a reified gay thing. This is Jeremy's experience.

Jeremy grew up in Charleston, South Carolina. His father, an alcoholic, was very critical of any glint of girlish behavior in Jeremy whose watchful eye was trained on differences between boy and girl activities. Jeremy envied certain girl activities but learned to monitor his gender-behavior closely, compulsively. He spent much of his adolescence in a state of hypervigilant self-scrutiny. The worst times he experienced occurred when his father got drunk watching TV. Jeremy would be called into the den, and his father, sloppy drunk, sentimental, and seemingly forgiving, would hug Jeremy, pull him into his lap and rock him like a baby declaring all the while, "I luv you Jeremy." Jeremy wanted to dissolve: this was not love, not love for Jeremy at least. As Jeremy grew older, he found that he could disguise this feeling (which he calls "low self-esteem") by having a buff body and a honed wit: "I am the Chelsea Queen you see before you today!" he reports somewhat sarcastically.

The dissolving experience was reiterated when Jeremy smoked crack. The call to the dealer and the stride to the ATM were "me operating without being present," Jeremy says. Though Jeremy has lost any sense of power, he holds together a look of strength. He jokes with the dealer (whose greed he ignores) and returns home. The dealer's job is to play dumb, to pretend that Jeremy is his homeboy. Back in his own space, shame and shyness overtake Jeremy. He has no blinds, so he crawls around the floor of his apartment gathering his paraphernalia. He smokes on the floor, slumped in a corner, and he imagines that he will be caught. He tries to blot out that feeling with the memory of a web site he visited just before picking up. It advertised unsafe sex parties. Its power was awesome to Jeremy who couldn't get out of his mind the wish to dissolve. He focuses on a feeling of connecting with the other "queens" in the extreme ad. Sometimes, he gets up the nerve to answer the ad, and he joins them in an obliterating orgy.

I had seen Jeremy around the neighborhood. A handsome, professional, seems to have it all Chelsea Boy. Then I saw Jeremy the day after his admission to a gay and lesbian affirmative inpatient psychiatric unit: skinny, moping, at a loss. He didn't recognize me at first. When he did, he confided in me, "I don't know if this gay unit is for me. I have nothing in common with these people. They don't know what it's like to be me." Jeremy profited from inpatient treatment in a gay specific context, as many severely addicted gay men do, largely because his peers quickly demonstrated that they did know what *it* was like to be him. Perhaps they weren't all as hip, urban or well educated. But they had all had troubles, and they had all sought a way out in drug and alcohol use. Unlike friends who were able to curb their use (or regulate their mood and affect when not using), they had used desperately and selflessly to the point of requiring inpatient-level care. Like Jeremy, they landed in a gay treatment center.

It is helpful to think about inpatient treatment as an alternative kind of Chelsea space in Jeremy's path toward recovery. Neisen (1996) who argues that gay men experience shame due to heterosexism (1993) has documented the benefits of gay affirmative treatment for substance abusers. In Neisen's view, gay men and lesbians live in a hostile environment that induces a feeling that one must blame oneself for one's sexuality or the victimization suffered. A negative self-concept develops over years of hearing derogatory messages about homosexuality, and many gays and lesbians attack themselves in destructive patterns of behavior that include drinking, drug abuse and/or suicidal gesturing. Neisen notes that a victim mentality may arise in individuals who struggle with feelings of inadequacy and helplessness, and he associates the process of recovery from heterosexist victimization with that from sexual and physical abuse more generally.

Neisen believes that affirmation is the critical variable. For Neisen, gay and lesbian patients need to reframe the statements that they make about themselves: from, "I can't be what I am" to "I don't deserve to be ashamed for being gay . . . for being who I am." He and Amico (1997) advocate for the importance of gay affirmative programs in facilitating that transformation. I, too, have noticed how patients who fare poorly in general psychiatric contexts thrive in a gay specific treatment center. It is indeed helpful to replace negative self-schemas with gay-positive ones. But I would argue that more goes on here than cognitive restructuring. Reified gayness is met and, in some introductory way, reckoned with. The process begins with the very name of the space where treatment will ensue. Take "Pride Institute" as an example. Here, a familiar gay moniker is applied to the space where treatment occurs rather than to the individuals who inhabit treatment.

I want to argue strongly that gay treatment programs promote self-efficacy among people with severe addictions because the mission and space for treatment objectify themselves. By this I mean that "gay treatment" stands in the relation of thing to the individuals who would partake of it. "Addiction" is a thing too, but not a thing that sponsors self-discovery through recognition. The structure of hospitalization adds an important dimension because it concretely and spatially sends this message: you need to be in a space that is controlled by someone other than yourself but, like you, everyone in that space is gay. Once there, "gay treatment" frees therapist and patient from the need to be gay or straight in some essential way, allowing them to be gay in more subjective ways. So it seems, patients who admit themselves to gay and lesbian specific programs experience being objectified and being rendered individual at the same time: the locked door objectifies; the gay cohort, in this space at least, subjectifies. As Jeremy noted, patients "act out." They flirt, demand, hide and seek, and display their needs to one another. Notably, they do this without substances–among like patients in a space that is not only a container, but Gay. "Rehab" becomes a synonym for "everyone there knows what *it* is like to be me."

Several months after inpatient treatment, Jeremy reported: "I need to really believe I'm an addict." He made the transition to outpatient psychotherapy and struggled to stay close to a 12-step regimen: "I need to have no options other than to see myself for what I am." He contrasts Narcotics Anonymous and therapy like this: "Therapy is harder for me. At NA, I know that everyone is in the same boat. I can't hide from them because they all know me–whether they know me or not. I raise my hand and share and I start to tell my story. Therapy's tougher because it's a relationship. I have to stay with it even when I want to run. I want to blame my therapist when I feel like

I'm going to fail. I can't do that in NA." Psychotherapy is, for now, uncomfortably subjective. Jeremy still prefers to relate to others who feel like a thing–but, he hopes, in a healthier way that makes it possible for him to tell his story.

The routines of Narcotics Anonymous are important for Jeremy, as is the identity of "recovering addict." It is a different identity than the reified sexual one he struggles with, but it is recognizable among peers in a similarly reassuring way. Different aspects of Jeremy's self-experience are in play here. Being an addict represents Jeremy's behavior but not his deeper "flaws." For Jeremy, addict behaviors have no subjective motive other than continuing use. Recognizing himself in the words of a speaker at a 12-step meeting returns a sense of dignity despite having done things that addicts do. The feelings and behaviors that Jeremy calls "flaws" are more personal. They summon desires. Think about Jeremy's phrase, "going where I have no business going" (above, when he described hooking up for unsafe sex on the Internet). We can interpret this literally: it is addict behavior to go there. On another level, it can also mean, "being what I have no business being, where I am not allowed to be, where I am flawed for wanting to go." When he was younger, Jeremy's father prohibited him from sitting in his armchair (there were many such prohibitions). Jeremy never questioned his father's rule; he worried that if he sat on the chair, he might sit like a girl.

In this context, "Going where I have no business going" could also mean, "I go to a place that is disallowed, but I go there by my own will." It has a sound of recognition in it: "perhaps I go to places that are bad for me on purpose?" Also, it is presumed that Jeremy and I both understand this. In this telling, "going where I have no business going" is a way of saying, "I can tell you that I have done something that I regret–even though I couldn't help myself." Jeremy is not simply sloughing off responsibility for his desire, he seeks to share it with someone whom, he perceives, gets it. The rapport is tenuous, however. Jeremy remains at great risk for relapse when he loses confidence in the connection and feels the wish to dissolve.

In Bollas' essay, Cruising in the Homosexual Arena (1992), he argues that cruisers struggle to master a sense of the erasure of self by "finding an erotic victim into whom this loss of control can be passed" (p. 154). He describes how isolated, "like an it," the child feels in the space of a mother whose confused need for the boy to be an extension of her make her into an "intimate stranger." The gay boy doesn't really know what he is to his mother or father: "this child cannot be his parent's boy, and is unsure if he can be his own person" (p. 156). He seeks to repair himself in "it-to-it" encounters with hot men who are ideal boys: "this alter being that possesses lost parts of the self is the object of intense need, the objectification of anguishing loss and, when it is acted out with the other, of a most ironic envy and hate."

Does the Chelsea Boy seek an erotic victim into whom his loss of control can be passed? Is Chelsea Boy substance use always malignant in Bollas' sense? Or may it also foster recognition and intersubjectivity? There are many possible outcomes when gay men meet other gay men who share a similar encounter with objectification and reification. The dynamic that Bollas and many others describe where it-to-it encounters repair problematic object relations may hold true in many cases (as it seems to with Jeremy), but it is an incomplete picture. It does not account for the possibility that the gay child is tangling with something other than the caretaker's subjectivity. As one patient told me, "I realized I was ashamed of the relationship I had with my mother and there was this whole other sissy thing happening." To overlook the importance of the child's encounter with politicized, objectified aspects of his fledgling identity limits our view of the broader course of his development. The overlap between developmental dramas and the encounter with reified categories of experience needs greater elaboration because it suggests that "it-to-it" relations are variable, not straightforward.

I have been arguing toward a broader, less tragic view of the space where reification and recognition meet. The process of becoming gay or male in a subjective way entails finding secure interpersonal space *and* dealing with the reified gay thing. Others who also feel something personal and political at the newsstand help us sort out life's confusing spectacles. In Chelsea space, I believe, it is recognition, not erasure, of the other that is sought–though, particularly in the depersonalizing context of addiction, it may not be found on the first outing.

NOTES

1. This image appeared on the cover of *The Adovcate*, May 25, 1999, which featured a special report on gay-transgender relations.

2. Chelsea became, in the late 1990s, the center of gay male life in New York. The neighborhood, whose main thoroughfare is Eighth Avenue, is home to many of the City's leading gay bars, clubs and gyms. I am using the term "Chelsea Boy" in lieu of the older term "clone" or the more specific current term "circuit boy" because it is a moniker that is used loosely and, typically, with a certain irony. Outside of New York, other names that describe objectified gay identity apply. I will use the name "Chelsea Boy" because it finds its way into mass media representations of urban gay men and, so, has broader use.

3. I will present a very abbreviated discussion of Marxist and psychoanalytic theories of reification and identification here in the interest of a focus on substance use practices that may be understood in the context of reification. A fuller theoretical discussion is forthcoming.

4. For more discussion of the "performative" aspect of identification, see Butler (1990).

5. For a witty spin on this much visited place, see Smith Galtney, Picked Last, OUT, Issue 71, October 1999, p. 58.

6. In Masud Kahn (1979) for example, the other in whom the "pervert" recognizes himself is not a person but a transitional object with whom one can only share a kind of engineered, intellectualized sexuality. While this type of object relation may characterize many people with profound addictions, I am arguing that it is not a sufficient account of the work that takes place in processes of recognition and identification.

7. Urbach (1996) provides a rich interpretation of the closet as a spatial relation one has with self and others.

8. In order to focus on addiction, I am deferring a discussion of reification and the sexual intimacy. I think that one could argue that many commonplace practices among gay men that have been linked to perversion or 'part-object" object-relations could be depathologized if understood within this framework.

REFERENCES

Amico, J. and Neisen, J.A. (1997), Sharing the secret: the need for gay specific treatment. *The Counselor*, May-June.

Benjamin, J. (1998), *Like Subjects, Love Object. Essays on Recognition and Sexual Difference*. New Haven: Yale University Press.

Bollas, C. (1987), *The Shadow of the Object: Psychoanalysis of the Unknown Thought*. New York: Columbia University Press.

_____ (1992), *Being A Character: Psychoanalysis and Self Experience*. New York: Hill and Wang.

Butler, J. (1990), *Gender Trouble: Feminism and the Subversion of Identity*. New York: Routledge.

Frommer, M.S. (1994), Homosexuality and psychoanalysis: technical considerations revisited. *Psychoanalytic Dialogues*, 4, 215-234.

Fuss, D. (1991), *Inside/Out*. In D. Fuss, ed., *Inside/Out*. New York: Routledge.

Hartman, S. (1995), Narrative Style/Narrated Identity. Resistances to categories of gay identity in the coming out story. Unpublished doctoral dissertation, New School for Social Research.

Hollinghurst, A. (1998), *The Spell*. New York: Viking.

Isay, R. (1989), *Being Homosexual*. New York: Avalon.

Lukacs, G. (1971), *Reification and the consciousness of the proletariate*. In, *History and Class Consciousness*. Cambridge, MA: MIT Press.

Masud Kahn, M.R. (1979), *Alienation in Perversions*. London: The Hogarth Press.

Mendelsohn, D. (1999), *The Elusive Embrace*. New York: Knopf.

Mitchell, J. (1982), *Introduction*. In, J. Mitchell and J. Rose, eds., *Feminine Sexuality: Jacques Lacan and the Ecole Freudienne*. New York: Pantheon, pp. 27-85.

Mitchell, S.A. (1993), *Hope and Dread in Psychoanalysis*. New York: Basic Books.

Neisen, J.A. (1993), Healing from cultural victimization: recovery from shame due to heterosexism. *Journal of Gay & Lesbian Psychotherapy*, 2:49-63.

_____ (1996), An inpatient psychoeducational group model for gay men and lesbians with alcohol and drug abuse problems. *Journal of Chemical Dependency Treatment*, vol. 7(3).

Urbach, H. (1996), Closets, Clothes, disClosure. *Assemblage* 30: 62-73.

Index

Abstinence
   celibacy as prerequisite, 114-116
   from methamphetamines, 113-114
Addicted professionals, 59-67
   personal memoir, 95-103
Addiction as learned behavior, 84-85
Adolescents, 69-80
   assessment, 72-75
   background and epidemiology,
     70-72
   treatment, 75-77
Affect theory, sexual compulsivity
     and, 142-147
AIDS. See HIV infection
AIM Project, 136-137
Alcoholics Anonymous (AA),
     14-16,91-92,100-101
   attitude toward gays, 14-15
   personal memoir, 95-103
   for teens, 76-77
Alcoholics Together, 14
Alcoholism, alienation and, 25-35
   background, 26-27
   discussion, 30-34
   literature review, 27-28
   method, 28-29
   results, 29-30
American Psychiatric Association,
     96,97,98
American Psychoanalytic Assocation,
     96
American Psychological Association,
     96,97
Amphetamines: MDMA
     (methylenedioxymethamphet-
     amine), 38,39-46
Amyl nitrate, 18
Anesthetics, as recreational drugs,
     46-49
Assessment

of adolescents, 72-75
   as part of treatment, 13-14,72-75
Association of Gay and Lesbian
     Psychiatrists, 98

Barebacking. See Risk-taking behavior
Biological co-factor models of
     treatment, 125
Bisexuality, 16,65-66

Calcium channel blockers, ketamine
     and, 48-49
Chelsea Boys, 169-185
Circuit parties, 18,19,37-57
   background, 38-39
   drugs used in, 39-52. See also
     specific drugs
   GHB (gamma-hydroxybutyrate),
     38,49-52
   ketamine, 38,46-49
   MDMA
     (methylenedioxymethamphet-
     amine), 38,39-46
Club drugs, 37-57. See also Circuit
     parties and specific drugs
     and drug types
Cocaine, 19
   crack, 105-122
Cognitive-behavioral approach, to
     sexual risk-taking and HIV
     infection, 134-138
Cognitive inhibition models of
     treatment, 124
Columbia University/The New York
     State Psychiatric Institute,
     37-57
Coming out, 89-90
Common underlying vulnerability
     models of treatment, 124-125

© 2000 by The Haworth Press, Inc. All rights reserved.

Contracts, 76,79-80
Crack cocaine, 105-122
Crank. *See* Amphetamines;
    Methamphetamine
Crystal meth. *See* Amphetamines;
    Methamphetamine
Cultural expectations, 16-17

Dean Alienation Scale, 28-35
Denial, 11,60
Depression: personal memoir, 95-103
Developmental issues, 9-13
Difference, psychology of, 10
Direct drug action models of
    treatment, 124
Dissociation, 11
Dopaminergic system, MDMA and,
    42-44
DSM-III, 97
DSM-IV, 142

Ecstasy. *See* GHB
    (gamma-hydroxybutyrate)
Effeminacy, 17
Epidemiology, 6-7
Ex-gay movement, 170

Family attitudes, 10-11,71
Family work with teens, 77
William J. Farley Center
    (Williamsburg, VA), 59-67

Gamma-aminobutyric acid (GABA),
    50
Gay males
    addicted professionals, 59-67
    of color, 18-19,63-64
    cultural expectations and, 16-17
    Jungian perspective on sexual
        compulsivity, 141-167
    older, 20
    perceived as effeminate, 17
    sexuality and, 90-91
    substance use issues specific to,
        16-20
    relationship life cycles, 20
    sexual activity, 19-20
    social life, 18-19
    types and patterns of substances
        used, 17-18
GBH. *See* GHB
    (gamma-hydroxybutyrate)
Genetic factors, 8
Georgetown University Medical
    Center, 81-94
Georgia State University, 25-35
GHB (gamma-hydroxybutyrate),
    38,49-52
    general properties, 49-50
    history, 50
    mechanism of action, 51-52
    psychological effects, 50-51
    treatment, 52
Gilgamesh (epic), 154-156
Green, Richard (author), 96-97
Growth hormone, GHB and, 51-52
Guilt, 91

Heterosexism. *See* Homophobia
History taking, 74-75
HIV infection
    as related to addiction, 87
    sexual risk-taking and, 123-139
        background and principles of
            treatment, 124-126
        cognitive-behavioral approach,
            134-138
        psychoanalytical approach,
            126-134
    sought by street teens, 20
    specialized programs and, 87-88
Home contracts, 76,79-80
Homophobia
    among professionals, 95-96,101-102
    as causative factor, 8-9
    internalized, 5-20
    specialized programs and, 85,89-90

Homophobic violence, 15
*Homosexual Behavior: A Modern
     Reappraisal* (Marmor), 97
Homosexuality in Perspective
     (Masters & Johnson), 98
Homosexual orientation, 7-8

Identity development, 9,11-12

Jungian perspective on sexual
     compulsivity, 141-167

Ketamine, 38,46-49
     general properties, 46
     history, 46-47
     mechanism of action, 48-49
     physiological effects, 47-48
     treatment, 49
"K hole" state, 48
Kinsey Rating Scale, 28

Lambda Center program, 81-94
     coming out and homophobia, 89-90
     conclusion, 92-93
     history of specialized programs, 84-85
     options in, 87-88
     social issues in recovery, 90-91
     spirituality and homosexuality,
         91-92
     structure of, 85-87
Lesbians. *See also* Women
     addicted professionals, 59-67
     alienation and alcoholism, 25-35
     substance use issues specific to, 16
Liquid ecstasy. *See* GHB
         (gamma-hydroxybutyrate)
Loyola Addiction Medicine Program
     (LAMP), 123-139

Major Depressive Disorder, 83
Maleness, cultural expectations of,
     16-17

MDMA (methylenedioxymetham-
         phetamine), 38,39-46
     general properties, 39-40
     history, 40-41
     mechanism of action, 42-44
     neurotoxicity, 44-45
     physiological effects, 41-42
     treatment, 45-46
Men, gay. *See* Gay males
Methamphetamine, 18,105-122
     appeal to gay men, 107-110
     celibacy and abstinence, 114-116
     clinical presentation of addiction,
         111-113
     establishment of early abstinence,
         113-114
     MDMA (methylenedioxymetham-
         phetamine), 38,39-46
     relapse fantasies, 119-120
     therapeutic approaches, 116-118
(University of) Michigan, 69-80
Michigan Alcoholism Screening Test,
     28-35
Models of treatment
     biological co-factor, 125
     cognitive inhibition, 124
     common underlying vulnerability,
         124-125
     direct drug action, 124

Narcotics Anonymous (NA), 14-16. *See
     also* Twelve-step programs
     for teens, 76-77
National Lesbian Health Care Survey,
     27
Neuroleptic Malignant Syndrome, 43,45
Neurotoxicity of MDMA, 44-45
New York University, 169-185
New York University School of
     Medicine, 105-122
NMDA receptors. ketamine and, 48-49
Numinous concept, 149-152
Nurses, addicted, 61-62

Older gay men, 20

Parental attitudes, 10-11,71
PCP, as compared with ketamine, 46-47
Physical examination, 74
Physicians
    addicted, 62-67
    personal memoir, 95-103
Political-psychological convergence,
    169-185
Poppers. *See* Amyl nitrate; Inhalable
    drugs
Post Hallucinogenic Perceptive
    Disorder, 44
Predisposition to substance use
    disorders, 7-13
PRIDE Institute, 84
Professional attitudes, 88
Professionals, addicted, 59-67,95-103
Psychiatric history, 74
Psychoanalytical approach to sexual
    risk-taking and HIV
    infection, 126-134
Psychoanalytic theory, 7-8,169-185
*(The) Psychoanalytic Theory of Male
    Homosexuality* (Lewes), 1
Psychology of difference, 10
Psychopolitical space, 169-185

Racism, 18-19
"Rave" culture, 37-57. *See also*
    Circuit parties
Recovery, 14-16. *See also* Treatment
    social issues in, 90-91
Recreational drugs. *See* Circuit parties
    *and specific drugs and drug
    types*
Reification, 169-185
Relapse fantasies, 119-120
Relationships, 20
    lesbian as compared with
        heterosexual, 33-34
Risk-taking behavior
    background and principles of
        treatment, 124-126
    cognitive-behavioral approach,
        134-138

psychoanalytical approach,
    126-134

San Mateo Mental Health Services,
    5-20
Screening instruments, 75
Serotonin, MDMA and, 39-40,42-45
Serotonin Syndrome, 43,45
Sex clubs, 19-20
Sexual activity, 19-20
    and affect of excitement, 145-147
    as displacement of affect, 147
    as release of suppressed affect,
        144-145
    as sedative, 143-144
Sexual addiction/sexual compulsivity,
    105-122
    classification from affect theory
        perspective, 142-147
    clinical case discussions, 156-165
    definition, 142
    epic of *Gilgamesh* and, 154-156
    Jungian perspective on, 141-167
    numinous and, 149-152
    shame as contributing to, 152-154
    teleological approach to treatment,
        147-149
Sexual Addicts Anonymous, 146-147
Sexual Compulsives Anonymous,
    146-147
Sexual history, 75
Sexuality, 90-91
    drug-fueled, 105-122. *See also*
        Methamphetamine
    linking with substance abuse, 12
Sexual risk-taking and HIV infection,
    123-139
    background and principles of
        treatment, 124-126
    cognitive-behavioral approach,
        134-138
    psychoanalytical approach,
        126-134
Shame, 91
    sexual compulsivity and, 152-154

(The) "Sissy-Boy Syndrome" and the Development of Homosexuality, 96-97
Social change, 8
Social history, 74
Social issues in recovery, 90-91
Specialized programs
  coming out and homophobia, 89-90
  conclusion, 92-93
  history of, 84-85
  options in, 87-88
  social issues in recovery, 90-91
  spirituality and homosexuality, 91-92
  structure of, 85-87
Special populations
  addicted professionals, 59-67
  adolescents, 69-80
Speed. *See* Amphetamines;
    Methamphetamine
Spirituality, 91-92,146-147
Subjectivity, 169-185
Substance use disorders
  epidemiology, 6-7
  issues specific to gay men, 16-20
  issues specific to lesbians, 16
  predisposition to, 7-13
  special psychotherapeutic
      considerations, 13-16
Substance use history, 74
Super K/Special K. *See* Ketamine
Symptom-relieving aspects, 12
Szasz, Thomas, 98

Teens. *See* Adolescents
Teleological approach to treatment of
    sexual addiction, 147-149
Transgender persons, as addicted
    professionals, 59-67
Treatment
  of adolescents, 75-77
  assessment, 13-14,72-75
  in drug-fueled sexuality, 105-122
  gay-sensitive, 13
  for lesbians specifically, 33
  lifestyle and related issues, 15-17

models of
  biological co-factor, 125
  cognitive inhibition, 124
  common underlying
      vulnerability, 124-125
  direct drug action, 124
  of sexual addiction, 147-149
sexual risk-taking and HIV
    infection, 123-139
  background and principles,
      124-126
  cognitive-behavioral approach,
      134-138
  psychoanalytical approach,
      126-134
special considerations, 13-16
specialized programs, 81-94
  coming out and homophobia,
      89-90
  conclusion, 92-93
  history of, 84-85
  options in, 87-88
  social issues in recovery, 90-91
  spirituality and homosexuality,
      91-92
  structure of, 85-87
of stimulant addiction, 116-118
twelve-step programs in, 14-16
Twelve-step programs, 14-16,91-92,
    100-101
  for addicted professionals, 59-67
  sexual addiction and, 146-147
  for teens, 76-77

University of Michigan, 69-80

Violence, homophobic, 15

Whitman Walker Clinic, 85-86. *See
    also* Specialized programs
William J. Farley Center
    (Williamsburg, VA), 59-67
Women. *See also* Lesbians
  alienation and alcoholism in lesbian
      and heterosexual, 25-35

SUNY BROCKPORT

3 2815 00840 0296

RC 564 .5 .G39 A33 2000

Addictions in the gay and
lesbian community

DATE DUE

APR 0 9 2003 ILL		
APR 1 7 2003		
AUG 2 7 2003		
SEP 0 7 2003		
DEC 1 3 2007		
NOV 1 2 2007		
MAY 1 7 2013		
APR 2 9 2013		

DRAKE MEMORIAL LIBRARY
WITHDRAWN
THE COLLEGE AT BROCKPORT

GAYLORD | | | PRINTED IN U.S.A.